Contributors

Julia Addington-Hall PhD
Lecturer in Health Services Research, Department of Epidemiology and Public Health, University College London Medical School , 1–19 Torrington Place, London WC1E 6BT

Sally Derry RGN RM
Matron/Centre Manager, Warren Pearl Marie Curie Centre, 911–913 Warwick Road, Solihull, West Midlands B91 3ER

Derek Doyle OBE FRCS(Ed) FRCP(Ed) FRCGP
7 Kaimes Road, Edinburgh EH12 6JR; formerly: Medical Director/Consultant Physician, St Colomba's Hospice, Challenger Lodge, 15 Boswall Road, Edinburgh EH5 3RW

Ilora Finlay MB DCH MRCGP
Consultant in Palliative Medicine, Velindre NHS Trust, Cardiff; and Medical Director, Holme Tower Marie Curie Centre, Bridgeman Road, Penarth CF6 2AW

Christopher Glynn MB MSc FRCA
Consultant and Honorary Senior Lecturer, Oxford Regional Pain Relief Unit, University of Oxford, Nuffield Department of Anaesthetics, Churchill Hospital, Headington, Oxford OX3 7LJ

Robert VH Jones MB BChir FRCGP
Honorary Senior Lecturer, Department of General Practice, University of Exeter, Foxenholes, Couchill Lane, Seaton, Devon EX12 2JH

Barbara Monroe BA BPhil CQSW
Director of Social Work, St Christopher's Hospice, 51–59 Lawrie Park Road, Sydenham, London SE26 6DZ

Ciaran O'Boyle PhD
Professor of Psychology, Royal College of Surgeons in Ireland Medical School, The Mercer Building, Mercer Street Lower, Dublin 2, Ireland

Charles D Shee MD FRCP
Consultant Chest Physician, Queen Mary's Sidcup NHS Trust, Frognal, Sidcup, Kent DA14 6LT; and Medical Adviser, Bexley Macmillam Team

naging illness

...nference organised
...on

Edited by
Gillian Ford CB FRCP
Medical Director, Marie Curie Cancer Care

and
Ian Lewin MD FRCP
*Consultant Physician, North Devon District Hospital,
Barnstaple, Devon*

ROYAL COLLEGE OF PHYSICIANS OF LONDON

1996

The Royal College of Physicians acknowledges
the financial support of this publication by
Marie Curie Cancer Care

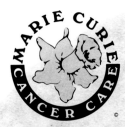

Royal College of Physicians of London
11 St Andrews Place, London NW1 4LE
Registered Charity No 210508

Designed and typeset by the Royal College of Physicians Publications Unit

Printed in Great Britain by Cathedral Print Services Ltd, Salisbury

Editors' Introduction

"Do I have to be dying before somebody will listen to me?"

"If only I'd known my mother-in-law had advanced cancer — all those lovely services".

Two remarks made more than a decade ago emphasise some perceptions about specialist palliative and hospice care: that the art of listening and communicating was not prominent in medical practice in Britain and that all the exciting development to support and care for people in their own homes or in specially designed in-patient units was limited to those who were dying from cancer.

Has the situation changed now? The growth in specialist palliative services in the past two decades, including the recognition of a medical specialty, palliative medicine, is evidence that principles and practice in this field are popular with the public and professions — and politically acceptable too. The challenge of the specialist services, 70 per cent of which are in the voluntary sector, is not to the NHS as an organisation, nor is it to do with funding, purchasing, or other financial issues. It is an approach to people which endeavours to see patients as members of a family, families as part of a community, the last days, weeks or months of life as valuable and as worthy of attention as any other part. The approach acknowledges issues of control and choice and seeks to weld the health professionals involved into a multi-skilled team bound by mutual respect and shared objectives.

But such patient-centred principles and practice are not, and should not be, confined to the specialty of palliative care. They can be woven into the whole fabric of clinical care, especially in the management of severe, prolonged or terminal disease — they are all the more necessary at a time when there is a temptation for care to become mechanistic and technology orientated. They are, in fact, relevant wherever people and families are grappling with diseases and conditions which can only be modified and alleviated but not cured.

The RCP Conference in May 1995, whose papers form the text of this book, was therefore planned to emphasise the needs of patients (and families) with diseases other than cancer. The overwhelming conclusion of the day was that patients with late stage incurable diseases, whatever the diagnosis, have needs which are not being met whether they are at home or in hospital. These needs require the same attention to detail and research that has characterised the approach to those with late stage cancer.

Doctors of course vary in their attitude to palliative care, and their personal vision will affect the way in which they make it available to their patients. Derek Doyle, in *Chapter 1*, describes the unmet educational and emotional needs of doctors which, if satisfied, would have a beneficial effect on the quality of care they provide. Charles Shee, in *Chapter 2*, and Sally Ann Derry, in *Chapter 3*, illustrate the relevance of a palliative care approach to severe respiratory and cardiac failure.

There may be many chronic conditions for which provision of care is suboptimal. This was confirmed by Robert Jones who describes, in *Chapter 4*, a survey of patients with Parkinson's disease, their families and carers. This theme is developed further by Julia Addington-Hall, in *Chapter 5*, who suggests that lessons from cancer care can point the way to improvements in the management of heart disease and stroke.

Pain, a common symptom in cancer, is often a major problem in those with non-malignant disease, and the success of treatment may hinge on this more than any other issue. Chris Glynn, in *Chapter 6*, describes his own approach to the physical and emotional aspects of pain control. Particular aspects of care must ultimately be judged by the individual patient, according to the ways in which they confer personal benefit. Professor Ciaran O'Boyle, in a College lecture which forms *Chapter 7*, explored complexities of measuring Quality of Life and presented a new way of doing this, which emphasises that individuals own their quality of life, not the observers or even the carers.

Palliative care services are still largely directed towards the patients with cancer, their families and carers. Yet the skills of the palliative care team, as described in *Chapters 8* and *9*, by Ilora Finlay and Barbara Monroe, are highly relevant and readily transferrable to the breadth of medical care.

This book is relevant to doctors, nurses, clinical psychologists, social workers, and other healthcare workers in hospital and community practice. We hope it conveys the realism, enthusiasm and commitment which came over at the symposium.

June 1996   GILLIAN FORD

                                                   IAN LEWIN

Contents

Acknowledgment   ii

Contributors   iii

Editors' Introduction   v

1. **What doctors are saying about palliative care**
   by Derek Doyle   1
   The meaning of palliative care to doctors   1
   Palliative care and the GP   2
   Educational approach to palliative care   4
   Conclusion   5
   References   5

2. **Managing late stage respiratory disease**
   by Charles Shee   7
   Medical treatment of COAD   7
   Pulmonary rehabilitation   8
   Support for people with severe respiratory disease   9
   Conclusion   10
   References   10

3. **Palliative care principles and terminal heart disease**
   by Sally Ann Derry   13
   Case history   13
   Symptoms of severe heart failure   14
   Medical management of severe heart failure   15
   Principles of palliative care and severe heart failure   16
   Psychological aspects   16
   Social aspects   16
   Spiritual aspects   17
   Conclusion   17
   References   17

4. **Palliative care and general practice**
   by Robert VH Jones   19
   Historical note   19
   Parkinson's disease as a model for palliative care   20

Boundaries and interfaces   22
References   23

5. **Heart disease and stroke: lessons from cancer care**

   by Julia Addington-Hall   25
   The Regional Study of Care for the Dying   25
      Group characteristics   27
   Symptom control   28
   Psychological support   30
      Awareness of prognosis   30
   Conclusions   31
   References   32

6. **Pain control in non-malignant disease**

   by Christopher Glynn   33
   An approach to pain management   33
   Quality of life and management of pain   34
   Palliative care   36
   References   36

7. **Quality of life in palliative care***

   by Ciaran O'Boyle   37
   The concept of quality of life   37
   QoL and palliative care   37
   Measuring QoL in palliative care   38
   QoL in palliative care: the need for an individual perspective   39
   QoL measures incorporating the individual perspective   41
   The Schedule for Evaluation of Individual QoL (SEIQoL)   42
   What DO SEIQoL studies tell us about Qol?   42
   First application of the SEIQoL in palliative care   44
   Some directions for future research   45
      Psychological models   45
      Social models   45
   Phenomenology and health-related QoL   46
   Acknowledgements   47
   References   47

* Royal College of Physicians Lecture delivered on 24 May 1995

8. Palliative care services: cancer and beyond
by Ilora Finlay   51
  Development of an outreach service   51
    Codes of practice   52
  Ethical decision making   52
  Children and parents   53
  Conclusion   54
  References   54

9. Terminal illness and the family
by Barbara Monroe   55
  Impact of terminal illness on the family   55
  Meeting the family   56
  Assessing need   57
  Talking with families   58
  Children   58
  Bereavement care   59
  Improving and extending palliative care   60
  Conclusion   61
  References   62

Marie Curie Cancer Care — its aims and work   63

1 What doctors are saying about palliative care

Derek Doyle

Medical Director/Consultant Physician, St Columba's Hospice, Edinburgh

Palliative medicine has been recognized as a sub-specialty in medicine only since 1987. It is concerned with the study and management of patients with active, progressive, advanced disease, in whom the prognosis is limited and where the focus is on quality of life. Whilst it certainly includes terminal care, it is concerned with far more than the final days or weeks of life.

The meaning of *palliative care* to doctors

The term *palliative care* means different things to different people. Some senior and junior doctors, when asked what it meant to them, gave me a variety of interesting replies, and here are some of them:

> '... *just a fancy name for terminal care, isn't it?*
>
> ... *de-luxe care for cancer patients*
>
> ... *mainly morphine as far as I can see*
>
> ... *we don't do it here; we either cure them all or send them to the hospice*
>
> ... *best left to those experts in the hospice*
>
> ... *I thought it was only for cancer patients but today I've referred three chest and heart patients*
>
> ... *I leave it to my junior staff; they've much more time than I have*
>
> ... *what we GPs do all the time*
>
> ... *the most difficult, demanding and delicate part of any doctor's work*
>
> ... *I'm only a houseman but it seems the most important thing I do; it's so rewarding*
>
> ... *I never took it seriously at medical school and now I do it every day; I feel so inadequate*
>
> ... *terribly important; I just wish I had some training in it* '

These replies show a range of understanding about the definition of palliative care. They also indicate the challenges and rewards, as well as the unmet educational and emotional needs at a professional level. The view that palliative care is synonymous with cancer care is understandable. There is public awareness of the spectrum of suffering in malignancy and the benefits of specialist care in dealing with such symptoms as pain, nausea, vomiting and breathlessness. In hospice and specialist palliative care units in the UK, 95% of in-patients have malignant disease. Even so, an increasing number of patients referred within hospitals to palliative medicine specialists have non-malignant disease.

Palliative care and the GP

Palliative care might be considered from three angles: the palliative approach, palliative techniques or procedures, and specialist palliative medicine.

Palliative care is the relief of pain and suffering, and the restoration of comfort, when cure is impossible or not an objective. It is an integral part of all medical care, whatever the underlying pathology or stage of illness. The fundamental principles are widely accepted (Table 1) and apply not only to cancer but equally to advanced cardiac, respiratory, neurological and HIV disease. What differentiates cancer care from, for example, geriatric care, is not the principle but the prevalence of issues (Table 2).[1]

Palliative techniques, designed to relieve symptoms, include a wide range of procedures, some of which are highly specialised. Examples include debulking of tumours by surgeons, radiotherapists or oncologists, stabilisation of cancerous bones by orthopaedic surgeons, fashioning of ostomies by general surgeons, and insertion of stents by urologists and chest surgeons.

Specialist palliative medicine is provided, for a minority of patients with special needs, by experts who have undergone higher professional training and accreditation. Specialist palliative care is currently provided by four main systems:

- domiciliary advisory teams which assist and support primary care teams;

- hospital palliative care advisory teams (support teams);[2]

- designated wards in general hospitals or cancer units;

- specialist units sited at hospitals, or independently, such as many hospices.

Table 1. The fundamental principles of palliative medicine.

Pain and symptom control
Psychosocial support
Spiritual support
Support of relatives
Multi-professional care

Table 2. Palliation problems in the terminal phase for geriatric and cancer patients.

	Geriatric patients (%)	Cancer patients (%)
Pain	25	75
Breathlesness	83	35
Constipation	50	80
Agitation	37	15
Communication difficulties	74	10
No visitors	20	5

GPs are, and need to be, deeply involved in palliative care. 90% of the last year of life is spent at home, 90% of the problems which need palliation arise at home, and 90% of the caring is done by relatives many of whom may themselves be elderly or frail.[3,4] With increasing awareness that the vast majority of palliative care could take place at home it seems inevitable that GP involvement will increase. In a general practice study, 29% of deaths occurred at home, about the urban average for the UK which, incidentally, is falling by 1% per annum. 40% of the deaths occurred in general hospitals and 31% in chronic care units. It was suggested that, with better provision of palliative care, 65% could have remained at home to die.[5] Another study, looking at the 40% who died in hospital, felt that admission was precipitated in three quarters of them by the need to relieve avoidable suffering and family strain.[6] There is still some ambivalence about the degree to which GPs should become involved in the logical extention of palliative care, which takes in the needs of the family. In one study, although a quarter of GPs felt that family care was important, an equal number thought it was not.[4]

There is some dissatisfaction with the current provision of palliative care in the community.[4,7-9] One study considered 65% of patients to have inadequate symptom control and another found 34% critical of their care, although 24% were grateful.[7] A study from one general practice looked at 85 deaths which had occurred in one year. Palliative care would have been feasible for the 50 deaths which were expected, where half the cases had malignant disease. Of these 50 cases, 39 died in hospital and 11 at home. Concern over provision of care and communication was expressed by relatives in 8 of 34 cases, and by the GPs themselves in 8 of the 50 cases.[8]

Educational approach to palliative care

Greater awareness, understanding, and the development of special skills will assure increasing quality of palliative care. An expert report in 1992 emphasised the importance of improved education at undergraduate and postgraduate levels in medicine, and in basic and post-basic education to diploma standard in nursing.[10] The recent increase in hospital based support services has provided a welcome means by which high quality palliative care can be extended to an increasing number of patients. At the same time it has provided an educational opportunity for doctors and nurses. Certainly, GPs and hospital doctors are aware of gaps in their training and seem keen to fill them (Table 3).[11]

Table 3. The perceived needs of GPs and consultants for further training in palliative medicine: a study of 300 Scottish doctors.

	GPs (Yes %)	Consultants (Yes %)
Would you consider it worthwhile working in an SPCU* for 4 weeks?	56	37
Would you attend special courses on:		
Physical caring	86	70
Emotional caring	83	69
Bereavement counselling	63	62

* Specialist Palliative Care Unit

Conclusion

The majority of doctors clearly recognize their responsibility to provide palliative care and few simply resort to automatic referral to a hospice. There is evident need for greater provision of palliative care, which would also allow people with terminal illness to spend more time at home. The quality of care is still variable and there is a tendency, in both general and hospital practice, for palliative care to be offered only at times of crisis. Anticipation and timely planning are essential for good management. Combined with educational opportunities and wise use of resources, this approach should assure an increasing standard of palliative care to a widening spectrum of patients.

References

1. Wilson JA, Lawson PM, Smith RG. The treatment of terminally ill geriatric patients. *Palliative Medicine* 1987; **1**: 149–53.

2. Haines A, Booroff A. Terminal care at home: perspective from general practice. *British Medical Journal,* **292**: 1051–3.

3. Levy B, Sclare AB. Fatal illness in general practice. *Journal of the Royal College of General Practitioners* 1976; **26**: 303–7.

4. Cartwright A. Changes in life and care in the year before death. *Journal of Public Health Medicine* 1981; **13**: 81–7.

5. Loven D, Goldberg E, Hart Y, Klein B. Place of death of cancer patients in Israel: the experience of a 'home care' programme. *Palliative Medicine* 1990; **4**: 299–304.

6. Herd EB. Terminal care in a semi-rural area. *Journal of the Royal College of General Practitioners* 1990; **40**: 248–51.

7. Sykes NP, Pearson SE, Chell S. Quality of care of the terminally ill: the carer's perspective. *Palliative Medicine* 1992; **6**: 227–36.

8. Blyth AC. Audit of terminal care in a general practice. *British Medical Journal* 1991; **330**: 983–6.

9. Dunphy KP, Amesbury BDW. A comparison of hospice and home care patients: patterns of referral, patient characteristics and predictors of place of death. *Palliative Medicine* 1990; **4**: 105–11.

10. Standing Medical Advisory Committee and Standing Nursing and Midwifery Advisory Committee. The Principles and Provision of Palliative Care. London: HMSO, 1992.

11. Doyle D. Education in palliative medicine and pain therapy: an overview. In Twycross RG (ed). The Edinburgh symposium on pain control and medical education, 1989. Royal Society of Medicine International Congress and Symposium Series, No 149.

2 Managing late stage respiratory disease

Charles Shee

Consultant Chest Physician, Queen Mary's Sidcup NHS Trust and Medical Adviser, Bexley Macmillan Team

Chronic respiratory disease is a distressing condition and causes 13% of adult disability in the UK. The major cause of chronic respiratory disease is chronic obstructive airways disease (COAD) ie chronic obstructive bronchitis and emphysema. It affects about 5% of men and 3% of women in middle age, and accounts for 1% of all hospital discharges in the UK and 5% of all deaths.[1] Tobacco smoking is a major cause of COAD and this is a worldwide problem. Sadly, as health campaigns lead to a decline in smoking in developed countries, tobacco companies are marketing increasingly in the Third World.

Medical treatment of COAD

Of the various pulmonary function tests used to monitor disease progression in chronic lung disease, the forced expired volume in one second (FEV1) is commonly used and convenient. Because of the non-linear relationship between lung function tests and disability, a small fall in FEV1 may result in a disproportionate loss of exercise capacity. The FEV1, which declines slowly with age, falls more rapidly in smokers than in non-smokers or ex-smokers. It is therefore never too late for those with significant COAD to stop smoking.

Drug treatments play an important role in COAD, although their effects tend to be disappointingly small in advanced disease. Inhaled bronchodilators are the mainstay of medical treatment. In contrast to asthma, anti-cholinergic inhalers, such as ipratropium or oxitropium bromide, may be more effective than beta-receptor agonists like salbutamol or terbutaline. In practice, many patients use both types of inhaler. Bronchodilators given by nebuliser are preferred by many patients with severe COAD, although they often have no advantage over delivery by an inhaler coupled to a spacer device. Antibiotics are frequently prescribed for exacerbations of COAD, often with little objective evidence of efficacy. Methylxanthines, such as theophylline, have some bronchodilator effect but there is a narrow window between therapeutic and toxic plasma levels.

The role of inhaled steroids in COAD is unclear, although they are the cornerstone of treatment for asthma. It is difficult to predict the minority who will respond to oral corticosteroids so all patients should have at least one formal trial of oral steroids to identify those with potential for reversibility.

For advanced COAD with severe hypoxia, long-term oxygen is the only intervention, apart from stopping smoking, likely to improve long-term survival, although the effect on quality of life may only be small.[2,3] Criteria for eligibility have been defined by the Department of Health and chest physicians are able to assess for eligibility and determine correct oxygen flow rates for each patient. In the UK, long-term domiciliary oxygen is usually provided via an oxygen concentrator. These can be prescribed by a chest physician in Scotland but only by GPs in England and Wales.

Pulmonary rehabilitation

Severe COAD is associated with considerable psychological and social morbidity. There is reduced quality of life with regard to physical and social functioning, mental health, pain perception and sleep, all of which correlate only poorly with lung function tests.[4,5] Dyspnoea is one of the most obtrusive symptoms and this can be aggravated by stress, anxiety, isolation and non-respiratory problems. Drug treatment for this specific symptom is rather unsatisfactory.[6,7]

A vicious circle may arise whereby depression, sense of loss, and low self-esteem all worsen the perception of dyspnoea. This leads in turn to inactivity, unfitness, further depression and isolation. Uncertainties over prognosis may also impose severe strain on family or carers. Patients often need encouragement and permission to exercise to breathlessness, and by experiencing dyspnoea in a medically controlled environment, they may overcome the anxiety and apprehension associated with it. Assuming that drug treatment for airways obstruction is maximised, pulmonary rehabilitation may help to break this vicious circle. Programmes of varying duration and complexity have been widely used in the USA since the 1970s, but there are still relatively few centres offering this facility in the UK.

The aim of pulmonary rehabilitation is to enable patients to attain maximum functional capacity.[8-10] This is achieved by a multi-disciplinary team through education, exercise, training, physiotherapy and psychotherapy. Most teams include a doctor, physio-therapist, pharmacist, social worker or psychologist, and a dietician. While there is usually little or no change in spirometry, arterial blood gases, rate of decline in FEV1 or prolongation of life, almost all studies have shown an improvement in exercise endurance, probably by improving mood and reducing the subjective perception of breathlessness.[10] Other benefits of rehabilitation include better quality of life [9,10] and possibly fewer hospital admissions.

Unanswered questions remain, and few studies have compared the effects of pulmonary rehabilitation with satisfactory control groups. It is important to know which components of these multi-disciplinary programmes are the most effective, the minimum intervention which is necessary, and the duration of any benefits.

Support for people with severe respiratory disease

It is important not to write off patients with respiratory failure caused by respiratory muscle weakness as in muscular dystrophy or previous poliomyelitis or as a consequence of severe chest wall disease, such as scoliosis or old thoracoplasty. A variety of positive and negative pressure devices are available for domiciliary respiratory support which can improve quality of life and reduce mortality.[11] Such cases, along with people with late stage interstitial lung disease, such as fibrosing alveolitis, are usually under frequent expert review. Patients with end-stage cystic fibrosis are usually under the care of specialist centres a few of which have their own domiciliary support teams.

Many people with COAD feel unsupported and there is some truth in this. A chest clinic study, looking at 160 people with severe disability from lung disease, found that only 6 were visited by a home help and only 3 by community or district nurses.[12] The British Thoracic Society recommends that there should be one respiratory specialist nurse in each Health District, but this target has not yet been achieved. In the UK respiratory specialist nurses are usually based in hospitals but a major part of their work is in the community. Their invaluable service for asthma, tuberculosis and lung cancer is well recognised, and patients and relatives appreciate their visits. However, for COAD, they have given limited measurable benefit in terms of preventing morbidity.[13]

Breathe Easy, a postal club set up by the British Lung Foundation, can be contacted at 8 Peterborough Mews, London SE6 3BL, by people who prefer this method of obtaining support and relieving their feelings of isolation.

Palliative care is concerned with the treatment of patients with disease that is active, progressive, far advanced and with a limited prognosis. Patients with advanced COAD and severe hypoxia fall into this category in that the majority will be dead within three years if not given long-term oxygen.[2] This prognosis, from time of first hospital admission, can be worse than for those with metastatic carcinoma of the breast or prostate. The course of the disease may be less predictable than that of some cancers as patients may go from one crisis to another over some years before a fairly rapid final event over a period of days.

Some hospices are precluded by charter from admitting terminally ill patients with non-malignant disease.[14] Others are prepared to do so and admit respiratory patients, partly to relieve the burden on families and home carers. If this practice of caring for advanced non-malignant disease is to develop, hospices will need a substantial increase in resources.[14]

Conclusion

For people with COAD, most of their last years of life are spent at home. Stopping smoking, medication, pulmonary rehabilitation and domiciliary oxygen may increase quality and quantity of life. It is probably inappropriate for palliative medicine specialists to take over their continuing care. However, it is highly desirable that principles of good palliative care should be applied, especially to improve home and community support. This is a worthy challenge for GPs and chest physicians.

References

1. Anderson HR, Esmail A, Hollowell J, Littlejohns P, Strachan D. Lower respiratory disease. In: Stevens A, Raftery J (eds). *Health Care Assessment Volume 1*. Oxford: Radcliffe Medical Press, 1994; 256–340.

2. Medical Research Council oxygen working party. Long-term domiciliary oxygen therapy in chronic hypoxic cor pulmonale complicating chronic bronchitis and emphysema. *Lancet* 1981; i: 681–5.

3. Nocturnal oxygen therapy trial group. Continuous or nocturnal oxygen therapy in hypoxic chronic obstructive lung disease. *Annals of Internal Medicine* 1980; **93**: 391–8.

4. Curtis JR, Deyo RA, Hudson LD. Health-related quality of life among patients with chronic obstructive pulmonary disease. *Thorax* 1994; **49**: 162–70.

5. Morgan AD, Peck DF, Buchanan DR, McHardy GJR. Effects of attitudes

and beliefs on exercise tolerance in chronic bronchitis. *British Medical Journal* 1983; **286**: 171–3.

6. Burdon JGW, Pain MCF, Rubinfeld AR, Nana A. Chronic lung disease and the perception of breathlessness: a clinical perspective. *European Respiratory Journal* 1994; **7**: 1342–9.

7. Shee CD. Palliation in chronic respiratory disease. *Palliative Medicine* 1995; **9**: 3–12.

8. Petty TL. Pulmonary rehabilitation in chronic respiratory insufficiency. 1: Pulmonary rehabilitation in perspective. Historical roots, present status, and future projections. *Thorax* 1993; **48**: 855–62.

9. Casaburi R, Petty TL (eds). Principles and practice of pulmonary rehabilitation. Philadelphia: WB Saunders, 1993.

10. Belman MJ. Pulmonary rehabilitation in chronic respiratory insufficiency. 2: Exercise in patients with chronic obstructive pulmonary disease. *Thorax* 1993; **48**: 936–46.

11 Simonds AK. Sleep studies of respiratory function and home respiratory support. *British Medical Journal* 1994; **309**: 35–40.

12. Waterhouse JC, Harper R, Marsh F, Jones NMB, Brazier J, Howard P. Quality of life in chronic airflow limitation. *Thorax* 1994; **49**: 417.

13. Littlejohns P, Baveystock CM, Parnell H, Jones PW. Randomised controlled trial of the effectiveness of a respiratory health worker in reducing impairment, disability and handicap due to chronic airflow limitation. *Thorax* 1991; **46**: 559–64.

14. Wilson IM, Bunting JS, Curnow RN, Knock J. The need for inpatient palliative care facilities for non-cancer patients in the Thames Valley. *Palliative Medicine* 1995; **9**: 13–8.

3 Palliative care principles and terminal heart disease

Sally Ann Derry
Matron/Centre Director, Warren Pearl Marie Curie Centre, Solihull

Heart failure is common, affecting about 1% of the population.[1] Definitions usually focus on the abnormality which prevents the heart from pumping blood at a rate commensurate with the metabolic requirements of tissues. Whilst true at a physiological level, this concept does not give a picture of how the patient is affected as a person. Yet good modern management of the patient with heart failure must also address psychological, social and spiritual issues using a holistic approach.

Case history

My personal realisation that principles of palliative care applied to the management of patients with severe heart disease occurred over 10 years ago. I was nursing a man with a dilated cardiomyopathy who had spent many weeks in our unit with severe, refractory heart failure. Although he was accepted for cardiac transplantation, a relatively new treatment at the time, he did not share our excitement and became increasingly difficult to manage. By chance, I was reading about the way in which principles of caring for those with advanced cancer could be used for any illness.[2] I was particularly interested in Elisabeth Kübler-Ross's description of the stages of loss often displayed by patients faced with the diagnosis of a terminal illness.[3] During the development of coping mechanisms they move through denial and anger to bargaining, depression and finally to acceptance.

We had so focused on the prospect of transplantation that we had failed to realise what this man's illness really meant. He was 32 years old, with a wife and 2 young children. He was too ill to work or even to accomplish the most basic self-care without help. His only chance of seeing another 12 months of life was to undergo a highly risky operation with no guarantee of success or even survival. Suddenly, it became transparently obvious that this young man was dying.

'The world rushes on over the strings of the
lingering heart making the music of sadness'

Rabindranath Tagore (Stray·Birds)

My textbooks had emphasised the value of open and honest communication with the terminally ill, the exploration of feelings and the process of encouraging emotions to be expressed. I did exactly what was recommended and asked him to tell me how he was feeling. More importantly, I listened to what he had to say. He told me he was very afraid and believed he was going to die. He wanted to sort out his affairs, make a will and spend time at home with his wife and children. After all, he might never see his home again. As a result of this, the first of many conversations, we were able to help him to achieve these important goals. Whilst we continued to manage his critical physical condition, we became much more aware of his need for psychosocial support. Interestingly, despite a steady worsening in his physical condition he became less angry and much easier to look after. He eventually received a heart transplant and lived for a further 7 years. I have always been grateful to him for teaching me such salutary lessons.

Symptoms of severe heart failure

Symptoms of severe heart failure are very similar to those of advanced cancer, with the exception of pain which is not a common feature. Poor ventricular function, resulting in fatigue and limited exercise tolerance, may frustrate any attempt to live an active life. Dyspnoea may be particularly distressing, sometimes occurring as paroxysms of pulmonary oedema at night, or causing a persistent cough. Oedema may first occur at the ankles but become more widespread with worsening myocardial function. This greatly increases the risk of pressure sores, whilst ascites may cause further discomfort. Hepatic congestion may give troublesome anorexia and nausea, symptoms which may also occur with digoxin intoxication. Jaundice may occur if the cardiac failure is intractable.

Other symptoms are also shared in common with neoplastic disease. Cachexia may initially be obscured by fluid retention although wasting may become evident in the limbs. Constipation may result from a combination of poor appetite, inactivity and drug treatment. Insomnia may show itself as a fear of going to sleep, or sudden arousal in panic with the development of pulmonary oedema. Sexual dysfunction, such as loss of libido or impotence, may add to feelings of worthlessness and depression.

Medical management of severe heart failure

Patients with severe chronic heart failure tend to be on a combination of drugs, sometimes at high dose, with the potential for adverse as well as good effects. Diuretics, whilst improving oedema, dyspnoea and fatigue, may cause troublesome gout, cramp and hyponatraemia. Angiotensin converting enzyme inhibitors improve the prognosis of cardiac failure[4-6] and they may improve the feeling of well-being, but they may also cause cough or aggravate hypotension. Additional treatments may be needed for angina, such as oral or transdermal nitrates. Calcium antagonists may be helpful but may have an adverse effect on myocardial function. Digoxin is of clear value in cardiac failure associated with atrial fibrillation and may confer some benefit in those in sinus rhythm. Other agents used to suppress abnormal rhythms may have the potential to cause others. The exact mixture of treatments therefore needs careful and expert adjustment, sometimes at frequent intervals.

Opioids have a valuable role in the management of severe heart failure. Diamorphine has welcome sedative and anxiolytic properties, and also decreases pulmonary venous pressure and the sensation of dyspnoea. Small doses are needed, 5–10mg of the elixir every 4 hours often being sufficient. Slow release morphine at a dose of 10–30mg twice daily is an alternative. In terminal heart failure a continuous subcutaneous infusion of diamorphine may be helpful, at a dose of 20–50mg over 24 hours.

In the presence of serious chronic illness, all symptoms, even those which seem relatively trivial, may assume major significance in the mind of the patient. They all need to be taken seriously and dealt with expediently. Anorexia and nausea may resolve with improvement in myocardial function, but anti-emetics, such as metoclopramide, may also be helpful, once digoxin toxicity has been considered and excluded. The mechanism of night cramps is not understood, but quinine sulphate, an effective treatment in many cases, should be used with caution in those with atrial fibrillation and heart block. Constipation is likely in those taking opioids so it should be prevented by the timely use of laxatives. If depression needs drug treatment, anti-depressants with low cardiotoxicity should be used by preference. Selective serotonin re-uptake inhibitors may be suitable.

Principles of palliative care and severe heart failure

When staged according to severity, rather like tumours, heart failure is easily perceived as a condition worthy of a palliative approach. The New York Heart Association classification defines 4 categories of heart failure:

- Class I: no limitation of physical activity;

- Class II: slight limitation of physical activity;

- Class III: marked limitation of physical activity; dyspnoea on mild exertion;

- Class IV: dyspnoea at rest.

For those with severe, Class IV, disease the 2 year mortality is almost 75%. In addition, about 50% of those with severe disease, and 20% of those with mild to moderate disease (Classes II-III) will require terminal care within one year of diagnosis.[1,6,7]

Psychological aspects

The psychological impact of heart disease is considerable. Many patients, notably those with ischaemic heart disease, may have come close to death on more than one occasion during the course of their illness. With worsening symptoms despite treatment, anxiety and fear may overwhelm both the patient and the family. The multiple losses resulting from such a disabling condition may give rise to feelings of regret and guilt about the past, and lead to anger most often aimed at those closest to the patient. Healthcare professionals may also find themselves a target of this anger because of their apparent failure to alter the course of events. This may be particularly so if the diagnosis and prognosis have not been discussed openly and honestly at an earlier stage. Acknowledging the feelings and helping the patient to understand and express them is likely to be more constructive than simply labelling the patient as difficult.

Social aspects

To really understand the effect of a life-threatening illness it is important to know what is going on at home. Drawing a family tree is a useful way of opening a discussion about who is at home, as well as offering the opportunity to talk about those who have left home or died. In the case of ischaemic heart disease, the family history may be very relevant to the way in which the illness is perceived by all concerned. Past losses still unresolved may compound the grieving process on which the patient and the family are currently embarked. Roles within the family may have been forced to change and this may have a marked effect on family dynamics, causing problems and conflict. The financial and housing implications of having someone chronically disabled living at home may well put additional strain on the whole family. Active listening is a powerful tool which helps the patient and family to identify problems, find solutions or agree compromises. This counselling process is often sufficiently supportive to enable them to cope at home for long periods.

Spiritual aspects

Faced with a loss of self-esteem, a lack of purpose, a sense of hopelessness, and the near death experience of pulmonary oedema, the patient with severe heart failure might experience a spiritual crisis. There may be a need to achieve peace of mind and to find meaning in a life almost over. There may be a need to love and be loved, to feel valued as a person, to forgive and achieve reconciliation. There may be a desire to rediscover or find God for the first time. Whilst there may be no easy answers to these issues, the counselling process may empower the patient to deal with the unfinished business and achieve realistic solutions.

Conclusion

Once underlying causes of heart failure have been corrected or improved, management is underpinned by the holistic principles of palliative care. Thus, plans for active and palliative care proceed in parallel. Control of symptoms and attention to psychological, social and spiritual concerns of both patient and family, can do much to improve the quality of life for all concerned.

References

1. Deedwania PC. Prevalence and prognosis of heart failure. *Cardiology Clinics* 1994; **12**: 1–9.

2. Saunders C, Baines M. Living with dying. The management of terminal disease. Oxford: Oxford University Press, 1989.

3. Kübler-Ross E. On death and dying. London: Routledge, 1990.

4. Davies MK. Congestive cardiac failure. Therapeutic progress review XXXIV. *Journal of Clinical Pharmacy and Therapeutics* 1989; **14**: 1–19.

5. The CONSENSUS Trial Study Group. Effects of enalapril on mortality in severe congestive heart failure. *New England Journal of Medicine* 1987; **316**: 1429–35.

6. The SOLVD Investigators. Effect of enalapril on survival in patients with reduced left ventricular ejection fractions and congestive heart failure. *New England Journal of Medicine* 1991; **325**: 293–302.

7. Cohn JN, Archibald DG, Ziesche S, Franciosa JA, *et al.* Effect of vasodilator therapy on mortality in chronic congestive heart failure. *New England Journal of Medicine* 1986; **314**: 1547–52.

4 Palliative care and general practice

Robert Jones

Honorary Senior Lecturer, Department of General Practice, University of Exeter

Amongst conditions commonly met in general practice some are self-limiting, some are curable, but many are incurable from the outset. Parkinson's disease, motor neurone disease, Alzheimer's disease, osteo- and rheumatoid arthritis are all examples of conditions which are not curable. There is an increasing awareness of the need for a palliative approach to such non-malignant, incurable conditions where the goal must be the best quality of life for patients and their families.[1] In this respect there is much common ground between general practice and specialist palliative care. How has this convergence come about? Consideration of the birth and early development of the College of General Practitioners and of the modern hospice movement show interesting parallels.

Historical note

The College of General Practitioners was established in November 1952 and by the mid 1960s a detailed statement concerning the knowledge skills and attitudes essential for general practice was clearly necessary. In 1969 a working party of the College defined the general practitioner as a doctor who provides personal primary and continuing medical care to individuals and families. His diagnosis would be composed in physical psychological and social terms, and he would intervene educationally preventively and therapeutically to provide for his patient's health.[2] At the same time Cicely Saunders had just founded St. Christopher's Hospice in London. Twycross has identified the main goals of hospice palliative care as to provide relief from pain and other distressing symptoms, to provide psychological care for the patient and for the family during the illness and in bereavement, and to provide a support system to help patients live as actively as possible in the face of impending death.[3] Both descriptions, accepted over 25 years ago, identified the need for the service to be personal, for diagnoses to be holistic and for the family and domestic carers to be included in the transaction.

A further similarity exists with regard to medical attitudes.

General practitioners are likely to have a primary interest in people, rather than specifically in their disease. On the same theme, the centre of interest for hospice care has shifted very much from the pathology to the person.[3] With such a history it is not surprising that general practice and the hospice movement have a common interest in the palliative approach.

Parkinson's disease as a model for palliative care

It needs to be asked whether people who have non-malignant incurable conditions really need the range of palliative care which includes physical, psychological, social and spiritual aspects as well as consideration of family carers. It will be useful to look at the needs of patients and carers drawn from a survey in which 521 people with Parkinson's disease and their 318 domestic carers were interviewed at home in South-West England in 1989–92.[4]

■ *Were symptoms recognised by doctors and nurses,*
  and were they relieved?

Of the 12 commonest symptoms volunteered to the interviewers by the 521 patients, 38% had not been noted in the history taken by a doctor or nurse (Table 1). Of the symptoms which had been discussed, fewer than half of those with dribbling, weakness, speech difficulty, worry, confusion, or depression had obtained relief. Clearly a need exists for better assessment and more effective palliation.

■ *Did patients have unrelieved psychological problems?*

Of those patients who were functionally independent, 29% were clinically anxious, as measured by the Hospital Anxiety and Depression scale (Table 2).[5] The proportion who were anxious rose to 42% amongst those with moderate functional deficit as measured by the Barthel ADL Index.[6] This indicates a high level of unmet need. Comparable figures applied to clinically significant depression.

■ *Were social problems addressed?*

Although few of the 318 carers thought they needed more domestic or financial help (about 8% in each case) increasing dependency and fear of leaving the patient had resulted in loss of social contact.

Table 1. The 12 commonest symptoms in 521 people with Parkinson's disease.

Symptom	Patients with symptom		Patients with symptom who had not told doctor/nurse		Patients who had obtained some symptom relief having told doctor/nurse	
	No	(%)	No	(%)	No	(%)
Loss of balance	366	(74)	107	(29)	129	(50)
Dribbling	292	(62)	134	(46)	67	(42)
Weakness	279	(54)	119	(43)	59	(37)
Speech difficulty	269	(52)	122	(45)	47	(32)
Constipation	266	(51)	49	(18)	198	(91)
Cramp	262	(50)	148	(56)	65	(57)
Dizziness	235	(45)	76	(32)	94	(59)
Worry	227	(44)	140	(62)	27	(31)
Pain	224	(43)	31	(14)	132	(68)
Confusion	211	(40)	131	(62)	13	(16)
Depression	209	(40)	122	(58)	32	(37)
Sleeping difficulty	209	(40)	62	(30)	96	(65)

Table 2. Anxiety and depression amongst 521 patients with Parkinson's disease by functional deficit.

Functional deficit	Anxious		Depressed	
	No	(%)	No	(%)
Independent (*n*=210)	60	(29)	39	(19)
Mild (*n*=183)	63	(34)	57	(31)
Moderate (*n*=77)	32	(42)	32	(42)
Severe (*n*=30)	12	(40)	14	(47)
Very severe (*n*=21)	6	(29)	7	(33)
Total (*n* = 521)	173	(33)	149	(29)

For example, although 75% of patients were functionally independent or only mildly affected, they would not be left by day by 37% of
carers, or at any time by a further 5%.

■ Were spiritual needs addressed?

Of the 190 patients who had previously attended a church regular-
ly, 105 had ceased to do so. Church visitors were involved with 75
patients, but a further 67, including some who had not previously
been regular churchgoers, would have liked to be visited.

■ Were the needs of family carers addressed?

Interviews produced no evidence of routine assessment of carers'
problems or quality of life by either hospital or general practice
staff. Most carers were over 65 years old and at least one major
clinical problem was suffered by 79% of males and 64% of females.
Many described themselves as tired, exhausted or frustrated, and
29% registered high strain levels on the Care Givers Strain Index.[7]
Yet few carers knew whether or not respite care was available in their
neighbourhood.

This brief review of service provision indicates that, although an
active palliative approach to care was needed, it was rarely available.

Boundaries and interfaces

With primary care taking place at home, and specialist secondary or
tertiary care taking place in hospitals, where do hospices fit in? They
certainly interface with primary care, frequently with secondary
care and occasionally with tertiary care. Different models of care
need to be applied according to the clinical circumstances.
Management of people with chronic incurable disease may occur
mainly within general practice with referral to specialists as appropriate. Alternatively, regular specialist review may take place mainly
within secondary care, or shared care might be appropriate using
agreed protocols. With hospices increasingly open to those with
non-malignant disease the options for service delivery becomes
more numerous.

Developments in nursing also affect the range of models available for providing care. Specialist nurses are increasing in number
and areas of interest. They may be based in a general practice, a
hospital or hospice, and their duties might be defined by geo-

graphical boundaries or by funding organisations such as national charities.

Although there is potential for much good, there is also the increasing possibility of confusion in management. Moreover, with regard to total care, quality of life and family involvement, there is little evidence as to comparative effectiveness, cost, or client preference for any of these multiple options.

There is a clear need for the palliative approach to be available to everyone with incurable conditions. At present the interfaces between providers of palliative care are frequently ill-defined and turbulent. Clarification depends on mutual understanding, goodwill and research.

References

1. The NHS Management Executive. *Circular EL(92)16.* 1992.

2. Royal College of General Practitioners. The educational needs of the future general practitioner. *Journal of the Royal College of General Practitioners* 1969; **18**: 358–60.

3. Twycross R. Hospice care. In Spilling R (ed). Terminal care at home. Oxford: Oxford University Press, 1986; 98.

4. Jones RVH. A Parkinson's Disease study in Devon and Cornwall. London: Parkinson's Disease Society, 1993.

5. Zigmond AS, Snarth RP. The hospital anxiety and depression scale. *Acta Psychiatrica Scandinavica* 1983; **67**: 361–70.

6. Cullin C, Wade DT, Davis S, Horce V. The Barthel ADL Index: a reliability study. *International Disability Studies* 1988; **10**: 61–3.

7. Robinson BC. Validation of Caregiver Strain Index. *Journal of Gerontology* 1983; **38**: 344–8.

5 Heart disease and stroke: lessons from cancer care

Julia Addington-Hall

Lecturer in Health Services Research, Department of Epidemiology and Public Health, University College London.

To date, developments in care for the dying and specialist palliative care services have focused almost entirely on cancer. This has over-shadowed the needs of the greater number of people dying from other diseases. Although an expert report in 1992 argued that palliative care services should be developed for patients dying from causes other than cancer,[1] little is known about the needs and the appropriate provision of service for such people. For example, although heart disease is the leading cause of death in the UK[2] a *Medline* search of papers published between 1983 and 1992 revealed no specific papers on the care of those dying from heart disease, but over a thousand on those dying from cancer. Management of dying and death are not well described in standard cardiological texts and there is also a lack of information on the care of those dying from other common conditions, such as stroke. More information on the needs and experiences of people dying from non-malignant diseases is needed if all dying patients, and their families, are to receive appropriate services, regardless of diagnosis.

In this paper, data from a population-based survey are used to compare the unmet needs of those dying from heart disease, the main cause of death in the UK, and those dying from stroke, who make up 13% of all UK deaths, with those dying from cancer.

The Regional Study of Care for the Dying

The *Regional Study of Care for the Dying* (RSCD) was established in 1990 to provide a contemporary account of dying and bereavement.[3] All district health authorities in England were invited to take part. Twenty agreed to do so, and although they were self-selected it seems likely that the survey results apply to the UK as a whole. The 20 districts covered inner city, outer urban and rural settings and were nationally representative on indicators of deprivation, death rates and health service provision.[4]

Survey methods were developed from those used by previous

studies.[5,6] Within each district a random sample was drawn from death certificates of residents dying in the last quarter of 1990. Most health authorities were particularly interested in people dying from malignancy, so cancer deaths were sampled disproportionately to ensure adequate numbers to evaluate care. Some ten months after the death a letter was sent to the usual address of the people who had died. It described the study and informed the recipient that an interviewer would soon make contact. The aim was to obtain information from family members and others who had known the deceased, and to interview them about events during the last year of life. Health problems, restrictions, sources of formal and informal help, the respondents' satisfaction with services, and their experiences of bereavement, were all to be examined. No attempt was made to distinguish between the terminal illness and other circumstances as causes of health problems or need for services.

A target was set of 200 completed interviews per district, to max-imise statistical confidence but limit the cost of the study. Altogether, 5375 letters were sent, and in 2915 cases (54%) there was a diagnosis of cancer. The response rate was 69%. Of the 3696 interviews, about a third (36%) were with the deceased's spouse, a similar number (35%) with a child or sibling, and the remainder were with more distant relatives (9%), friends or neighbours (9%), or officials (10%). The median time between the deceased's death and interview was 44 weeks, with an inter-quartile range of 40–50 weeks. There were some differences between the main causes of death of the interviewed sample and those for all adult deaths in England for 1990. Sex of the deceased did not differ from national data but age at death did. For those aged 55–64 years deaths were under-represented, whilst for those aged 75–84 years they were over-represented[3].

People who died suddenly without warning, premonitory illness or time for care, are excluded from the analyses presented here. The remaining sample comprises 2063 deaths from cancer, 683 from heart disease, and 229 from stroke. Three issues are addressed: firstly, whether people who die from heart disease and stroke need better symptom control in the last year of life; secondly, whether they need psychological support; and thirdly, whether they need more open communication with healthcare professionals about death and dying. Results for cancer deaths are included to put the results for heart disease and stroke into context. This helps to focus discussion on whether the current situation is appropriate, whereby cancer patients receive the bulk of specialist palliative services.[7]

Further details on the experiences and needs of people dying from cancer and stroke are also reported elsewhere.[8,9]

Group characteristics

As expected, cancer deaths occurred at an age that was younger than for either heart disease or stroke (Table 1).

Stroke deaths were particularly likely in the elderly. Such people were also more likely to have lived alone, to have been widowed, and to have died in nursing or residential homes. Appropriate patterns of services for those who die from stroke are therefore likely to be quite different from those who die from cancer. The emphasis should perhaps be less on home care and family support and more on trying to ensure high standards in nursing homes. However, those in both the stroke and heart disease groups who were under the age of 65 at death, married, or who died at home, might well need the sort of psychological and family support currently provided for people who are dying from cancer. Further research is

Table 1. Characteristics of 2975 deaths in the survey.

Diagnosis	Cancer (*n*=2063) %	Heart disease (*n*=683) %	Stroke (*n*=229) %
Age at death:			
<65	26	9	7
65–74	28	27	14
75–84	33	40	40
85+	13	23	39
Lived alone	31	38	44
Marital status:			
married	51	41	26
widowed	35	47	59
other	14	12	16
Place of death:			
own home	29	29	9
hospital	50	55	67
hospice	14	0	0
residential/nursing home	7	12	24
other place	0	4	0

needed to establish the proportion of people who die from stroke and heart disease who might benefit from such services.

Symptom control

Respondents were asked whether the deceased had suffered pain in the last year of life, to what degree it had been distressing, for how long it had been present, and whether it had been present in the last week of life (Table 2). The results indicate that, although pain is less common in patients with stroke and heart disease than in those with cancer, it is more likely to be be long-lasting and, in at least two fifths, it may cause considerable distress.

These results need cautious interpretation. Because of the study design, which was necessarily simple, we cannot assume that all reported pain was caused by the condition from which the patient died. Some pain was undoubtedly a result of other diseases, such as arthritis. The pain was also reported by respondents after the death of the patients. Their descriptions might have diverged from the views of the patients themselves, and they might have been affected by bereavement and the passage of time after death. Some evidence suggests reasonably good agreement between patients' and carers' assessments of physical symptoms[10,11] but the subject needs further investigation by prospective study.

Respondents were asked whether GPs and hospital doctors had provided satisfactory pain relief. The results show that cancer patients are not alone in needing improved pain control (Table 3).

A range of symptoms experienced in the last year of life, apart from pain, are shown in Table 4. Nausea and vomiting, difficulty swallowing and constipation are commonly associated with dying from cancer and, as expected, are less common in the heart disease

Table 2. Pain in the last year of life.

Report of pain	Cancer %	Heart disease %	Stroke %
in the last year of life	88	77	66
in the last week of life	67	63	48
for more than 6 months[1]	58	75	78
'very distressing'*	61	50	43

* Percentage of those who had symptom in last year of life.

and stroke groups. Control of breathlessness is a challenge in the palliative care of cancer patients and needs to be researched further.[12] The same may apply to the large numbers who die from heart disease each year, where this symptom is even more common.

Expertise in symptom control acquired with cancer patients may not necessarily transfer well to the care of people dying from other conditions, where the causes and natural history of symptoms are different. Given the different age profiles of the three groups, and the nature of their diseases, people dying from stroke were more likely to have mental confusion, and to have been incontinent. These symptoms are also likely to have lasted for more than six months in stroke patients. This suggests that the pattern of service provision for dying stroke patients should differ from that for cancer patients. The emphasis should be not so much on medical

Table 3. Respondents reporting that treatment by doctors relieved pain only partially or not at all.

	Cancer %	Heart disease %	Stroke %
General practitioners	47	50	49
hospital doctors	35	34	51

Table 4. Prevalence of symptoms other than pain in the last year of life.

	Cancer %	Heart disease %	Stroke %
Breathlessness	54	60	37
Nausea and vomiting	59	32	23
Difficulty swallowing	41	16	23
Constipation	63	38	45
Mental confusion	41	32	50
Pressure sores	28	11	20
Urinary incontinence	40	30	56
Bowel incontinence	32	17	37

interventions but more particularly on skilled nursing care to alleviate symptoms such as incontinence and pressure sores.

Psychological support

A majority of patients in all three groups were reported to have felt low at some point in the last year of life (Table 5). This symptom was commonest in cancer patients but it tended to be more prolonged in those with stroke or heart disease. Of those reported to feel low at some point, over three quarters of patients in the heart disease and stroke groups had this symptom for at least six months, compared with about half those with cancer. A high level of psychological morbidity has been found in other studies of stroke patients[13] and may be caused partly by the need to adjust to disability. This may also be true for some of the heart disease group.

Awareness of prognosis

Respondents were asked whether the patients were aware of the possibility of imminent death. Three quarters of those with cancer and almost half in the heart disease and stroke groups were believed to have known or suspected that they were likely to die soon. Although some were evidently told by health care professionals, just over 40% of cancer patients were thought to have worked this out for themselves, compared to twice as many in the stroke and heart disease groups (Table 6).

Respondents were also asked whether they knew or suspected imminent death. Excluding officials and healthcare workers, a fifth in the cancer group had realised for themselves compared to twice as many in the heart disease and stroke groups (Table 6).

Table 5. Patients reported to feel low or miserable in the last year of life.

	Cancer %	Heart disease %	Stroke %
last year of life	69	59	57
last week of life	47	42	33
for more than 6 months*	54	82	78
'very distressing'*	52	50	45

* Percentage of those who had symptom in last year of life.

Prognostic judgments may be difficult in all three of these disease categories. More knowledge is needed on what prognostic information is shared particularly with heart disease and stroke patients, what they would like to know, and what consequences arise from not knowing. Taken together these figures suggest that, for heart disease and stroke, the prognosis is given preferentially to relatives and carers rather than to the patient, a situation which prevailed in cancer care some years ago. Regarding help in dealing with issues of death, it seems likely that some patients with heart disease and stroke will have similar needs to those with cancer. The size of this group is not known but their needs might well be met by the frankness and expertise in counselling and support developed within palliative care.

Conclusions

Many who die from heart disease or stroke would benefit from a more palliative approach to their care. They need better symptom control, more psychological support and more open communication with healthcare professionals. For some, access to specialist palliative care might alleviate difficult symptoms. This might also give opportunity for expert counselling and support when patients and their families are trying to come to terms with dying.

Many questions about the needs of people dying from non-malignant diseases remain unanswered and accurate prognostic

Table 6. Awareness that the patient was going to die.

	Cancer %	Heart disease %	Stroke %
Patients			
Knew	76	49	40
Did not know	16	39	35
Unknown	8	12	25
Respondents			
Knew	77	37	57
Half knew	13	22	22
Did not know	11	41	22
Realised themselves			
Patients	42	81	80
Respondents	20	42	36

judgements may be difficult. It is certainly clear that cancer patients are not alone in needing symptom control, psychological support and open communication with healthcare professionals. Quality of care might also be enhanced if the palliative philosophy is applied to these patients well before it is absolutely clear that they are going to die.

References.

1. Standing Medical Advisory Committee and Standing Nursing and Midwifery Advisory Committee. The Principles and Provision of Palliative Care. London: HMSO, 1992.

2. Office of Population Censuses and Surveys. *1990 Mortality Statistics.* London; HMSO, 1991.

3. Addington-Hall JM, McCarthy M. The Regional Study of Care for the Dying: methods and sample characteristics. *Palliative Medicine* 1995; **9**: 13–8.

4. Addington-Hall JM, McCarthy M. Can national surveys be funded successfully from local NHS resources? Evidence from the RSCD. *Journal of Public Health Medicine* 1995; **17**: 161–3.

5. Cartwright A, Hockey L, Anderson JL. Life before death. London: Routledge and Kegan Paul, 1973.

6. Cartwright A, Seale C. The natural history of a survey: an account of the methodological issues encountered in a study of life before death, London; King's Fund, 1990.

7. Higginson I. Palliative care: a review of past changes and future trends. *Journal of Public Health Medicine* 1993; **15**: 3–8.

8. Addington-Hall JM, McCarthy M. Dying from cancer: results of a national population-based investigation. *Palliative Medicine* 1995; **9**: 295–305.

9. Addington-Hall JM, Lay M, Altmann D, McCarthy M. Symptom control, communication with health professionals and hospital care of stroke patients in the last year of life, as reported by surviving family, friends and carers. *Stroke* 1995; **26**: 2242–2248.

10. Higginson I, Priest P, McCarthy M. Are bereaved family members a valid proxy for a patient's assessment of dying? *Social Science Medicine* 1994; **38**: 553–7.

11. Field D, Douglas C, Jagger C, Dand P. Terminal illness: views of patients and their lay carers. *Palliative Medicine* 1995; **9**: 45–54.

12. Higginson I, McCarthy M. Measuring symptoms in terminal cancer: are pain and dyspnoea controlled? *Journal of the Royal Society of Medicine* 1989; **82**: 264–7.

13. Ebrahim S. Clinical Epidemiology of Stroke. Oxford: Oxford University Press, 1990.

6 Pain control in non-malignant disease

Christopher Glynn

Consultant and Honorary Senior Lecturer, Oxford Regional Pain Relief Unit, University of Oxford, Nuffield Department of Anaesthetics, Churchill Hospital, Oxford.

Pain is an unpleasant sensory and emotional experience associated with actual or potential tissue damage, or described in terms of such damage. In the treatment of chronic pain, both its components need to be addressed, the sensory or physical, and the emotional response. It should be distinguished from nociception, the response to a noxious stimulus.[1]

An approach to pain management

Each patient has a different constellation of pain, disability and expectations. Before treatment, patient and family or carers need to be clear about the aims, limitations and possible side effects of any therapy. If there is no definitive therapy for a cause of pain, this should be explained. When a patient is unable to communicate freely, as in Alzheimer's disease for example, the accurate assessment of pain may be difficult. Observations by the spouse, family members or carers need to be noted and incorporated into the plan of management. Vicarious feelings of distress, derived from their view of the patient's pain, need to be resolved by explanation, reassurance and adequate treatment. If any of the participants have a discrepant agenda, the end result will tend to be unsatisfactory.

There is no clear evidence of a change in either perception of pain or pain threshold with increasing age. However, there is a change in expectation of pain relief with age, and the elderly do not expect to be totally free from pain.[2] The effect of age on the emotional response to stress or chronic pain, has not been studied in detail. Emotional responses and coping mechanisms may or may not differ from the young.[3]

Control of chronic pain in terminal non-malignant disease can be divided into the definitive management of the cause of the pain, symptomatic management, or the palliative approaches. Guidelines for managing the physical component of chronic pain are summarised in Table 1. Definitions of neuropathic pain evidently suggest that treatment with narcotics is ineffective.[1] This is not entirely true. Morphine has been used successfully in all types of chronic pain and although this, and other narcotics, are less effective than some other treatments, they should always be given a trial for neuropathic pain.[4]

Broad guidelines for treatment of the emotional component of chronic pain are outlined in Table 2. Patients with chronic pain need to be reassured that an emotional response to pain is normal. Indeed, it is abnormal not to have an emotional response to chronic pain. Whether this response needs treatment will be a combined decision between the patient and the doctor. Referral to a psychologist or psychiatrist should only take place with the understanding and agreement of the patient.

Quality of life and management of pain

Patients with severe non-malignant disease, like those with cancer, are often concerned about quality more than quantity of life. Chronic pain may be perceived as a cause of diminished quality, and any treatment which reduces this further is likely to be unwelcome. Each patient should be dealt with individually and the first step is to

Table 1. Treatments for the physical component of pain.

Physical	Conventional	Physiotherapy TENS
	Unconventional	Acupuncture
Pharmacological	Conventional	Non-narcotic Narcotic
	Unconventional	Anticonvulsants Antidepressants Adrenergic blockers Alpha$_2$ agonists
Injections	Diagnostic	Somatic nervous system
	Therapeutic	Sympathetic nervous system
Operations	Definitive	for the cause of pain
	Symptomatic	for the management of pain

define that patient's understanding of what the pain means and his or her expectations of pain relief.

If there is a specific treatment for a cause of pain, its risks and benefits need to be discussed as they apply to that individual. An example might be a proposed hip replacement where there are risks of anaesthesia in someone with respiratory disease. For severe respiratory disease the risks of symptomatic pain management are far less than the risks of surgery. Results may not be as dramatic as if surgery were possible, but it is usually possible to improve chronic pain provided the patient's expectations are realistic.

In some situations, such as osteoporotic collapse of a vertebra, pain relief may lead to substantial increase in physical ability. However, in some cases, pain relief may not be followed by the improved quality of life which has been anticipated. Thus, the patient whose hip replacement does gives pain relief may find mobility equally restricted by concurrent cardiovascular or respiratory disease.

The relationship between chronic pain and quality of life and is not simple. Like pain, quality of life is an individual and subjective phenomenom. For each patient there are different meanings and expectations. As an illustration, patients were asked to report the effect of an epidural injection on pain and quality of life. The results were interesting. Quality of life was improved in 4 patients whose pain relief was less than two weeks, but not in 5 in whom it was greater than 12 weeks. It is obviously important to define patient's expectations of pain relief and what benefits might ensue. Some patients do not distinguish between pain and disability, both of which are unpleasant.

Table 2. Treatments for the emotional component of pain.

Pharmacological	*Conventional*	Antidepressants Anticonvulsants
	Unconventional	Narcotics Alternative medicine
Counselling	*Conventional*	Professional counsellor Psychologist Psychiatrist Cleric
	Unconventional	Faith healer

Pain is not always considered in the assessment of quality of life in the elderly. Specialised instruments designed to assess quality of life seem to overlook pain in the elderly,[5] even though it is common.

Palliative care

Patients with terminal non-malignant disease have the same physical and emotional problems with death and dying as those with malignant disease. The challenge to good care is highlighted by a prospective study of the terminal event in patients with chronic renal failure who elected to discontinue dialysis.[6] In this planned situation a comfortable and good death was frustrated in 4 of the 11 patients (36%) because of unresolved pain and agitation.

In terminal patients with cancer, morphine relieves pain in more than 80% of cases. It should be possible to provide similar pain relief for the majority of patients with terminal non-malignant disease using the same approach. If morphine is not effective, because of side effects or because the pain is not morphine sensitive, the pain clinic should be able to provide other therapies. The total relief of pain in all patients is probably not a realistic expectation, but success in more than 90% is achievable with the use of all facilities available. In the final stages of the disease it may also be important to involve physicians in palliative medicine. This is the message from Cohen *et al.*[6]

References

1. Merskey H, Bogduk N. Classification of chronic pain. Seattle: IASP Press, 1994.

2. Gibson SJ, Helme RD. Age differences in pain perception and report: a review of physiological, psychological, laboratory and clinical studies. *Pain Reviews* 1995; **2**: 111–37.

3. Melding P. How do older people respond to chronic pain? A review of coping with pain and illness in elders. *Pain Reviews* 1995; **2**: 65–75.

4. Jadad AR, Carroll D, Glynn CJ, Moore RA, McQuay HJ. Morphine responsiveness of chronic pain: double-blind randomised cross-over study with patient-controlled analgesia. *Lancet* 1992; **339**: 1367–71.

5. Fallowfield L. The quality of life in the elderly. In: Fallowfield L (ed). The quality of life, the missing measurement in health care. London: Souvenir Press, 1990; 162–85.

6. Cohen LM, McCrue JD, Germaine M, Kjellstrand CM. Dialysis discontinuation a 'good' death? *Archives of Internal Medicine* 1995; **155**: 42–7.

7 Quality of life in palliative care

Ciaran A O'Boyle

Professor of Psychology, Royal College of Surgeons in Ireland Medical School, Dublin

'If you really want to help somebody, first you must find him where he is. This is the secret of caring. If you cannot do that, it is only an illusion if you think you can help another human being. Helping somebody implies your understanding more than he does, but first of all you must understand what he understands.'

Kierkegaard, 1859.

The concept of quality of life

Quality of life (QoL) and the related concept of health status are becoming increasingly important in assessing the impact of disease, illness and treatment.[1-5] A search of *Medline* using the term QoL indicates that the annual number of publications in which the term is mentioned has increased from 8 in 1974 to 284 in 1984 and 1209 in 1994. The annual number of publications in which QoL was the central theme increased from 2 to 93 and 502 respectively, over the same periods. The importance of the QoL concept is that it places the patient at the heart of the therapeutic process. Methodologies derived to measure QoL offer the potential for a final common pathway for assessing the multidisciplinary inputs of basic scientists and clinicians to diagnostic and treatment processes.[6] QoL, therefore, could become the dominant criterion by which medical decisions are made and treatment advances are judged. However, the concepts underlying QoL are complex and multidimensional and this has resulted both in differing conceptualisations of QoL and a wide variety of measurement techniques which reflect the lack of agreement on definition.

QoL and palliative care

QoL is particularly relevant to people with far advanced terminal illness and concern with QoL is at the core of palliative care. Patients are people first and foremost; the sick and disabled are not merely biological substrates for treatment. Failure to acknowledge their QoL is neither good science nor good medicine. QoL is a multi-dimensional construct. It is designed to capture all the essential conditions beyond mere survival that have to be fulfilled if the chronically ill and dying are to experience meaning in their lives. Symptom control is obviously important but the great efforts in palliative care to control pain and manage symptoms serve a deeper existential purpose. They free a sick and dying person's time for acts and experiences meaningful and powerful enough to demonstrate 'that for a short moment there is no death and time does not unreel like a skein of yarn thrown into an abyss'.[7] Of course, palliative care is no longer reserved for those facing imminent death. Instead, it represents a multidisciplinary approach to the alleviation of suffering at any point in the disease trajectory.[6]

Despite the central importance of QoL in palliative care, it is only recently that research has been undertaken in this area.[8] Although many QoL methods have been developed for public health research and oncology, their use has been limited particularly in palliative care.[9] Where they have been used in this context, problems of theory and methodology have reduced the value of the research. For example, an important limitation of the US National Hospice Study was that QoL was rated solely by observers using the Spitzer Quality of Life Index and not by the patients.[10]

Measuring QoL in palliative care

There is a consensus that measurement of QoL in palliative care should be comprehensive. Evaluation should cover key domains such as physical symptoms, physical role and social functioning, psychological distress, cognitive function, body image and sexual function.[11] One approach to measurement is to adopt scales which were developed for oncology. These include the Spitzer Quality of Life Index,[12] the Functional Living Index — Cancer (FLIC),[13] the Rotterdam Symptom Checklist,[14] the Cancer Rehabilitation Evaluation Systems (CARES)[15] and the Functional Assessment of Cancer Treatment (FACT).[16] There are, however, several problems in applying generic oncology instruments to patients receiving palliative care.[8] Firstly, these measures do not adequately tap the relevant domains. The particular needs of terminally ill patients increase the significance of domains such as satisfaction with information and treatment, spirituality and existential considerations which must be addressed in any comprehensive scheme. Secondly, these measures focus excessively on physical symptoms which may bear little relationship to QoL in such patients. Finally, the orientation of many such measures is negative. They attempt to measure QoL by compiling a list of problems rather than by attempting to measure positive contributions to QoL.[17]

Some progress has been made in developing specific QoL scales for palliative care. MacAdam and Smith[18] developed a 43 item questionnaire which focused on the perceptions of patients receiving palliative care. Five factors were identified as being most important to patients: mood; gastrointestinal symptoms; fears and family worries; knowledge and involvement in treatment and support. Unfortunately, the questionnaire underwent little development beyond the initial stage. A questionnaire which attempts to combine generic and disease specific approaches has been developed by the European Organisation for Research and Treatment of Cancer (EORTC)[19] and a palliative care module is currently under development.[20] Recently, Cohen *et al*[17] have developed the McGill Quality of Life Questionnaire in a palliative care setting. It measures four constructs: physical symptoms, psychological symptoms, outlook on life, and meaningful existence which the authors consider to be particularly important. It differs from most other questionnaires in that the existential domain is measured, the physical domain is important but not predominant and positive contributions to QoL can be measured.

QoL in palliative care: the need for an individual perspective

'When it comes to saying in what happiness consists, opinions differ, and the account given by the generality of mankind is not at all like that of the wise. The former take it to be something obvious and familiar, like pleasure or money or eminence and there are various other views and often the same person actually changes his opinion. When he falls ill he says that it is his health, and when he is hard up he has that it is money.'

Aristotle (384–322BC) Ethica Nichomachea

When trying to relieve suffering in the dying it is particularly important to know which particular issues are of most concern to the patient at any given time. Only a dying person can judge their own experiences and they do so in the context of their own expectations, hopes and fears, philosophies and beliefs. Karl Rogers, a pioneer of the phenomenological approach in psychology said: 'the best vantage point for understanding behaviour is from the internal frame of reference of the individual himself'.[21] We have proposed a phenomenological approach to QoL. That is one which focuses on the individual's personal view of life and of its quality. We have suggested that QoL should be defined as what the individual determines it to be.[22,23] Similarly, Hayry[24] has proposed that 'the quality, or value, of an individual's life is no more and no less than what she considers it to be'. This approach, while acknowledging environmental influences on individual behaviour and perception, emphasises the central role of the individual in creating his or her world. Individuals are active agents, involved in a continuous search for meaning and constantly striving towards the goal of self-actualisation.

The importance of the individual perspective in medicine and healthcare has been stressed by others. Cohen [25] proposed that persons are best viewed as lives lived with some degree of coherence; a human person is a life lived according to a human plan. It is the plan of life and the inter-related purposes of a person that give his or her life its unity and meaning. When asked to say who we are, we reflect on our aims and upon the causes with which we identify. We give an account of ourselves when we say what we did, or are doing or intend to do with our lives. Features of human life can be judged by their effect on the life plan. QoL is, therefore, reflected in the capacity of the individual to realise his or her life plans. This view helps to explain why some features of human life are considered to be positive while others are considered to be negative. Intelligence, stamina, mobility and good health contribute to the realisation of human plans. Features of life such as pursuit of one's vocation, the practice of one's art, the enjoyment of one's special pleasures and talents are evidence that the plan is being advanced. Some qualities of human life, however, hinder or block the pursuit of a person's life plan: disease, confinement to bed or to an institution, mental instability, fear and pain. Based on this philosophy, improving the quality of a patient's life will involve attention to some elements which can be valued by everyone since they will tend to maximise the realisation of life plans. However, since experiences, ambitions and plans are individual, some elements will be of particular importance to particular patients. In any assessment of QoL it is necessary to assess these elements which the individual considers important.

Calman[26] proposed a similar view. Qol is the difference, at a particular point in time, between hopes and expectations and present realities. It depends upon past experience, present lifestyle and personal hopes and ambitions for the future. The gap between hope and reality may be narrowed by improved function through treatment or by reduced expectations through understanding the limitations imposed by the disease or by accepting the balance of risks and benefits which might be conferred by treatment.

QoL measures incorporating the individual perspective

'In every concrete individual, there is a uniqueness that defies all formulation. We can feel the touch of it and recognise its taste, so to speak, relishing or disliking, as the case may be, but we can give no ultimate account of it, and have in the end simply to admire the Creator.'

William James, 1912

Many authors have acknowledged the importance of the individual's perspective in rating QoL, but have doubted the possibility of assessing such individual concerns in a standardised manner. Clinical experience indicates that patients with serious illnesses, especially those who are terminally ill, engage in a search for personal meaning. Consequently, any measure of QoL in palliative care must reflect the patient's sense of personhood and meaning in life.

Instruments developed to measure QoL in cancer patients have usually been designed to monitor the impact of anti-cancer therapy during pre-palliative phases of the illness so they have limited application to palliative care. Even in the pre-palliative phase such questionnaires often fail to measure QoL and are more correctly considered as health status measures. Pre-defined lists of items must be rated by respondents in a particular manner, whether they are personally relevant or not. Weights assigned to each answer are unlikely to represent the weights which the respondent would assign if given the choice. Measures such as these impose a value system which may not be that of the respondent.

Despite the difficulties, a number of QoL measures have been developed which incorporate the perspective of the individual patient.[27] Some of these may yet prove to be suitable for palliative care settings. Common to these measures is an attempt to assess functioning on those aspects of life which the respondent considers to be important. Measures such as the Anamnestic Comparative Self-Assessment,[28] Quality of Life Index (QLI),[29] measures based on the Repertory Grid Technique[30,31] and the Patient Generated Index[32] all have potential applications in palliative care settings although modification may be necessary to reduce the burden on patients.

The Schedule for Evaluation of Individual QoL (SEIQoL)

We developed the Schedule for the Evaluation of Individual QoL (SEIQoL)[27,33,34] to measure three elements of QoL. In a structured interview, respondents nominate five areas of life (cues) which they consider most important to their overall quality of their life. For each area they rate their current status against a vertical visual analogue scale. This is labelled at the upper and lower extremities by the terms 'as good as could be' and 'as bad as could be', respectively. From the replies, the interviewer generates a profile using bar charts. The respondent is asked to consider the profile and rate their global QoL on a horizontal visual analogue scale. At this stage of the procedure, the interviewer knows which areas of life are most important to the respondent and the current status on each.

Judgment analysis is used to quantify the relative importance of each cue. The respondent is presented with 30 randomly generated profiles of hypothetical subjects labelled using their five previously chosen cues and asked to rate the global QoL for each profile. Unknown to the respondent, ten profiles are repeated in order to estimate the consistency of the judgments (internal reliability: r). The relative weight attached by the respondent to each cue in judging global QoL is calculated by multiple regression. The technique also generates a measure of the variance (R^2) in overall QoL judgements explained by the five cues used. This statistic provides an estimate of the internal validity of the respondent's judgments. The investigator can, therefore, assess how well the particular judgment policy models the individual's assessment of QoL (R^2) and also how reliably (r) judgments are made. A global QoL score is derived by multiplying the relevant cue weights by the individual's current self-rating and summing across the five cues. The SEIQoL, therefore, determines which the areas of life (cues) the respondent considers important, current functioning in each area, and the relative importance of each area together with indices of internal reliability and validity.

What do SEIQoL studies tell us about QoL?

Do nominated cues vary across individuals?

If QoL is a phenomenological construct, it will vary between individuals. One cannot assume that a particular area of life will be important to a particular individual. Our studies show that, whilst some cues like health, family and work, which are often assessed by standardised QoL measure are frequently elicited using the SEIQoL, other cues such as spirituality, finance and education are also nominated. Cues unique to a given individual such as politics, aesthetics and time left to live, are also elicited frequently. Types of cue, their permutations and combinations are many and varied. Patients with the same condition may generate very different profiles. For example, we found that cues nominated by patients who were HIV positive or who had AIDS varied as a function of their life situation. Whilst global scores indicated that gay men and intravenous drug users both had significantly lower QoL than a control group, the specific cues nominated by the two patient groups were quite different from each other.[35]

Are individuals consistent in their judgments of QoL?

Respondents making reliable judgments should rate consistently the overall QoL associated with the 10 repeated profiles. A range of studies indicated that individuals are generally consistent about their QoL judgments[33] and this is particularly true of palliative care patients.

Do individuals tend to nominate the same cues over time?

Particular aspects of life vary with time and changing circumstances. For example, a serious illness or a personal disaster might lead to a reassessment of the values to which one subscribes. Life might then be lived a moment at a time in order to extract as much enjoyment and meaning from it as possible.[36] It is important, therefore, when using patient generated ratings to determine how stable such ratings are over time.

In developing the SEIQoL we examined whether individuals nominate the same cues after an elapsed period of time. The stability of elicited cues was calculated from the mean number of cue changes for populations in which no intervention was made between interviews. In a range of healthy respondents, we found that domains which individuals judge to be important to their QoL are likely to remain relatively constant over periods as long as two years.[33]

What does the SEIQoL tell us about health-related QoL?

Many investigators feel that consideration of QoL in healthcare should be restricted to a sub-component of QoL called health-related QoL. Patrick and Erickson define health-related QoL as the value assigned to opportunity, perception, functional status impairment and death associated with events or conditions as influenced by disease, injuries, treatment or policy.[37] However, the phenomenological approach would suggest that this view is unnecessarily restrictive. Health, because of its enabling nature, is likely to influence many aspects of life, some of which may be relevant to only a small number of individuals. It is difficult to determine in advance which factors can be excluded when assessing health-related QoL from a phenomenological perspective. Any aspect of life considered important by the patient could be important in the evaluation of QoL in the context of health. Amongst the assumptions implicit in many current QoL measures is that everyone considers health to be important, that its relative importance invariably increases when one is unwell and that QoL automatically declines as a disease progresses. We have repeatedly found that health is not the most common cue mentioned by patients and that the relative weight assigned by those who do nominate it varies considerably from person to person and over time.[33] In this context, an interesting aspect of the McGill Quality of Life Questionnaire developed by Cohen *et al* has been the reduced emphasis on physical symptoms in assessing the QoL of patients receiving palliative care.[17]

First application of the SEIQoL in palliative care

Recently, 30 consecutive patients receiving palliative treatment for cancer completed the full SEIQoL and also a shorter direct weighting procedure.[38] They were all aware that their disease was at a palliative stage. The frequencies of cues nominated as being important to QoL were: family 93%; health 77%; spiritual life 47%; friendships 33%; finances 33% and social activities 27%. The very high validity (Mean R^2 = 0.84) and reliability outcomes (Mean r = 0.84) are the highest scores found in any SEIQoL study to date and suggest that patients receiving palliative care may have a particularly deep insight into their QoL and be particularly reliable in making QoL judgments. Whilst the SEIQoL was found to be acceptable in the palliative care setting, it is likely to be too complex for routine use. We have recently found that much simpler direct method of measuring cue weights is reliable and valid[27] and this is currently under investigation in palliative care.

Some directions for future research

Psychological models

Psychological models appropriate to palliative care need to be developed. One working hypothesis is that, as the patient approaches death, symptoms and physical factors become relatively less important and intrapsychic factors become relatively more important for patients. The phenomenological perspective recognises the dynamic nature of QoL and separates it from any external definition of health. A number of studies indicates that patients often report their QoL to be as high as that of a healthy group. These findings raise important questions about the cognitive construction of QoL; how this is maintained by individuals and in particular how such cognitive constructs adapt to changing circumstances. We need to know much more about how individuals adapt to major changes in their health. This is particularly important given the increasing use of advance directives or living wills[39] in which patients are asked to judge in advance the type of treatment they would wish based on a projected QoL in a terminal or vegetative state. Allied to this is the need to determine the congruence between QoL judgments made by a patient and those made by a proxy such as a carer.

There is a need for cross-sectional QoL studies focusing on describing the status of all patients in palliative care. Longitudinal studies are also needed to assess the effects of palliative care from initiation to the death of the patient. In the longer term, QoL measures are likely to contribute significantly to the process of audit and quality control. Both medical and non-medical interventions are important in palliative care and there is a growing need for randomised clinical trials to assess the impact of a range of treatments.

Social models

Illness has a different meaning for each person involved in the process, the clinician, nurse, family and patient. Each applies different criteria to judge illness severity and treatment efficacy. Doctors and nurses are more likely to use physiological indicators and symptom ratings while family members and patients are more likely to use QoL type assessments. In fact, QoL is a conceptual model intended to represent the perspective of the patient in quantifiable terms. It can be viewed as the final common pathway measure representing the net effect of the disease and all the medical and psychosocial therapies brought to bear from the perspective of the patient.[6] Patients with advanced cancer are often reported to rate the quality of their lives better than do observers and to make different choices about treatment than might be expected. Higginson and McCarthy[40] developed the Support Team Assessment Schedule (STAS) as a measure of outcome of palliative care from the perspective of the palliative care team. This was developed through comparisons with the views of patients and family members. Results showed particular differences between the ratings of the various observers and patients. Team members identified more problems than patients' self-ratings, except for pain control where team members identified fewer problems. Team members' ratings fell between those of the patient and the family members. Coates *et al* compared continuous and intermittent chemotherapy for advanced breast cancer.[41] Contrary to the expectations of the physicians, continuous chemotherapy was found to be superior to intermittent chemotherapy in improving the QoL of patients. In another study, patients with cancer were much more likely to opt for radical treatment with minimal chance of benefit than were people who did not have cancer, including medical and nursing professionals.[42] Research is needed to establish the factors which influence QoL judgments by proxy raters, be they healthcare professionals or others, particularly in view of the increasing use of proxy decision makers in determining clinical interventions.[39]

Phenomenology and health-related QoL

In health care, the phenomenological approach complements the increasing emphasis on patient autonomy and informed consent. Competent and autonomous patients need to, and will make health care decisions based, *inter alia,* on their evaluation of the implications for their QoL. Poor adherence to medical advice may result from patients making decisions based on their personal assessment of the therapeutic benefit of an interventionn against its negative effects, an assessment often related to their QoL. Such decisions by patients may be difficult for doctors to accept. Ideological struggles can occur between doctors, who adopt a rational objective approach to QoL, and patients who view QoL in terms of their unique personal situation. A doctor, assessing a patient and deciding which therapy is suitable, must analyse a host of individual variables. The approach to assessing individual QoL described here is not foreign to the manner in which good clinicians have always assessed and treated their patients. For clinicians, patients and families, individualised measures of quality of life may help to formulate treatment plans and monitor progress in terms most significant to the patient.

Patients are not passive recipients of fate. They are active, perceiving, thinking beings engaged continuously in pursuit of personal meaning. In the face of death, weighed down by symptoms, they can still struggle upward in a search for meaning and transcendence. Considerable suffering in one domain may be overridden by an enhanced sense of personal meaning in another resulting in a net increase in QoL despite coexisting suffering.[43] The measurement and management of symptoms, be they physical, psychological or social, is obviously important but by limiting our focus in this way we run the risk of missing the essence of QoL for patients receiving palliative care. If we are to understand a patient we must enter as fully as possible into his individual frame of reference. To use Kierkegard's term we must understand what he understands. This may be new and unfamiliar ground, requiring a different type of science, less concrete and technological perhaps but more human. The American psychologist Abraham Maslow once said that 'the value-free, value-neutral, value-avoiding model of science that we have inherited from physics, chemistry and astronomy where it was necessary and desirable to keep the data clean, is quite unsuitable for the scientific study of life'. One might add 'and death'

Acknowledgements

The research reported here was funded by grants from Ciba, The Irish Health Research Board, The Irish Department of Health and The Royal College of Surgeons in Ireland. Dr Waldron's research has been funded by a research grant from the Irish Hospice Foundation.

References

1. Spilker B (ed). Quality of life assessments. *In:* Clinical Trials. New York: Raven Press, 1990.

2. Walker SR, Rosser RM. Quality of life assessment: key issues for the 1990s. London: Kluwer Academic Press, 1993.

3. O'Boyle CA. Assessment of quality of life in surgery. *British Journal of Surgery* 1992; **79**: 395–8.

4. Bowling A. Measuring health: a review of quality of life measurement scales. Milton Keynes: Open University Press, 1991.

5. Bowling A. Measuring disease: a review of disease-specific quality of life measurement scales. Milton Keynes: Open University Press, 1995.

6. Schipper H. Quality of life: the final common pathway. *Journal of Palliative Care* 1992; **8(3)**: 5–7.

7. Roy DJ. Measurement in the service of compassion. *Journal of Palliative Care* 1992; **8(3)**: 3–4.

8. Roy DJ, Schipper H (eds). Quality of Life. *Journal of Palliative Care* 1992 ;**8(3)** (Special issue)

9. MacDonald N. Oncology and palliative care: the case for co-ordination. *Cancer Treatment Reviews* 1993; **19 (Supplement A)**: 29–41.

10. Morris JN, Suissa S, Sherwood S, Wright SM, Greer D. Last days: a study of the quality of life of terminally ill cancer patients. *Journal of Chronic Diseases* 1986; **39**: 47–62.

11. Cella DF. Quality of life: the concept. *Journal of Palliative Care* 1992; **8(3)**: 8–13.

12. Spitzer WO, Dobson AJ, Hall J, Chesterman E *et al.* Measuring the quality of life of cancer patients: a concise ql-index for use by physicians. *Journal of Chronic Diseases* 1981; **34**: 585–97.

13. Schipper H, Clinch J, McMurray A, Levitt M. Measuring the quality of life of cancer patients: the functional living index — cancer. Development and validation. *Journal of Clinical Oncology* 1984; **2**: 472–3.

14. deHaes I, Van Knippenberg FC, Neijt JP. Measuring psychological and physical distress in cancer patients: structure and application of the Rotterdam Symptom Checklist. *British Journal of Cancer* 1990; **62**: 1034–8.

15. Ganz P, Schag CA, Lee JJ, Sim MS. The CARES: a generic measure of health-related quality of life for patients with cancer. *Quality of Life Research* 1992; **1**: 19–29.

16. Cella DF, Jacobsen PB, Orav EJ, Holland JC *et al.* A brief POMS measures of distress for cancer patients. *Journal of Chronic Diseases* 1987; **40**: 939–42.

17. Cohen SR, Mount BM, Strobel MG, Bui F. The McGill quality of life questionnaire: a measure of quality of life appropriate for people with advanced disease. A preliminary study of validity and acceptability. *Palliative Medicine* 1995; **9**: 207–19.

18. MacAdam DB, Smith M. An initial assessment of suffering in terminal illness. *Palliative Medicine* 1987; **1**: 37–47.

19. Aaronson NK, Ahmedzai S, Bergman B, Bullinger M, *et al* for the EORTC Study Group on quality of life. The European Organization for Research and Treatment of Cancer QLC-30: a quality of life instrument for use in clinical trials in oncology. *Journal of the National Cancer Institute* 1993; **85**: 365–76.

20. Ahmedzai S. Quality of life measurement in palliative care: philosophy, science or pontification. *Progress in Palliative Care* 1993; **1**: 6–10.

21. Rogers CR. Client-centred therapy. Boston. Houghton Mifflin, 1951.

22. Joyce CRB. Quality of life: the state of the art in clinical assessment. In: Walker SR, Rosser RM (eds). Quality of life: assessment and application. Lancaster: MTP Press, 1988.

23. O'Boyle CA, McGee HM, Hickey A, O'Malley K, Joyce CRB. Individual quality of life in patients undergoing hip replacement. *Lancet* 1992; **339**: 1088–91.

24. Hayry M. Measuring the quality of life: why, how and what? *Theoretical Medicine* 1991; **12**: 97–116.

25. Cohen C. On the quality of life: some philosophical reflections. *Circulation* 1982; **66 (Supplement 3)**: 29–33.

26. Calman KC. Quality of life in cancer patients — an hypothesis. *Journal of Medical Ethics* 1984; **10**: 124–7.

27. O'Boyle CA. The schedule for the evaluation of individual quality of life. *International Journal of Mental Health* 1994; **23(3)**: 3–23.

28. Bernheim JL, Buyse M. The anamnestic comparative self-assessment for measuring the subjective quality of life of cancer patients. *Journal of Psychosocial Oncology* 1983; **1**: 25–38.

29. Ferrans CE, Powers MJ. Quality of life index: development and psychometric properties. *American Journal of Nursing Science* 1985; **8**: 15–24.

30. Thunedborg K, Allerup P, Bech P, Joyce CRB. Development of the repertory grid for measurement of individual quality of life in clinical trials. *International Journal of Methods in Psychiatric Research* 1993; **3**: 45–56.

31. Dunbar GC, Stoker MJ, Hodges TCP, Beaumont G. The development of SBQoL — a unique scale for measuring quality of life. *British Journal of Medical Economics* 1992; **2**: 65–74.

32. Ruta DA, Garratt AM, Leng M, Russell IT, McDonald LM. A new approach to the measurement of quality of life: the patient generated index. *Medical Care* 1994; **32**: 1109–26.

33. O'Boyle CA, McGee HM, Hickey A, Joyce CRB *et al*. The Schedule for the Evaluation of Individual Quality of Life. User manual. Dublin: Department of Psychology, Royal College of Surgeons in Ireland, 1993.

34. O'Boyle CA, McGee H, Joyce CRB. Quality of life: assessing the individual. In: Albrecth GL, Fitzpatrick R (eds). Quality of life in health care. *Advances in Medical Sociology*, 5. London: JAI Press, 1995, 159–80.

35. Hickey A, Bury G, O'Boyle CA, O'Kelly FD *et al*. Quality of life implications of infection with the human immunodeficiency virus. *Proceedings of the WONCA/SIMG Congress*. Brussels, 1993.

36. Taylor SE. Positive illusions: creative self-deception and the healthy mind. New York: Basic Books, 1989.

37. Patrick DL, Erickson P. Assessing health-related quality of life for clinical decision-making. In Walker SR, Rosser RM (eds). Quality of life assessment: key issues for the 1990s. London: Kluwer Academic Press, 1993; 11–64.

38. Waldron D, O'Boyle CA, Moriarty M, Kearney M, Carney D. Use of an individualised measure of quality of life; the SEIQoL in palliative care. Results of a pilot study. *Proceedings of the Palliative Care Research Forum.* Durham, 1995.

39. Advance directives. Editorial. *Lancet* 1992; **340**: 1321–2.

40. Higginson IJ, McCarthy M. Validity of the support team assessment schedule: do staffs' ratings reflect those made by patients or families. *Palliative Medicine* 1993; **7**: 219–28.

41. Coates A, Gebski V, Bishop JF, Jeal PN *et al.* Improving the quality of life during chemotherapy for advanced breast cancer. *New England Journal of Medicine* 1987; **317**: 1490–5.

42. Slevin ML, Stubbs L, Plant HJ, Wilson P *et al.* Attitudes to chemotherapy: comparing views of patients with cancer with those of doctors, nurses and general practitioners. *British Medical Journal* 1990; **300**: 1458–60.

43. Cohen SR, Mount BM. Quality of life in terminal illness: defining and measuring subjective well-being. *Journal of Palliative Care* 1992; **8(3)**: 40–5.

8 Palliative care services: cancer and beyond

Ilora Finlay
Consultant in Palliative Medicine, Velindre NHS Trust, Cardiff, and Medical Director, Holme Tower Marie Curie Centre, Penarth

Symptom control is a fundamental part of the palliative care team's work. Expertise developed in the field of cancer is now applied increasingly to symptom control in non-malignant disease. As with other units, the Cardiff team is particularly involved in the management of emotional distress and agitation, pain, emesis, intractable dyspnoea, constipation, wound and stoma care.

There is an increasing range of chronic, severe, non-malignant conditions where we are asked to take part in management. These include genetic diseases such as the muscular dystrophies and cystic fibrosis, neurological disease like motor neurone disease and multiple sclerosis, severe cardiorespiratory and rheumatoid disease, and many others.

Development of an outreach service

The outreach palliative care service which we have developed has extended the work of the Marie Curie Centre in Penarth. The need for this became evident in a survey at the University Hospital of Wales. It revealed potential for improvement in the quality of care of patients with cancer and other chronic disease. The service became possible when the cancer care charity's operating rules were modified to allow hospice access for patients with non-cancer diagnoses.

An active educational programme was started and simple guidelines were written for control of pain, nausea, vomiting and constipation. Collaboration with the pharmacy department helped to spread information about the service via the network of ward clinical pharmacists.[1] The survey was repeated two years later. It confirmed the positive impact of palliative medicine advice on prescribing and on quality of life of those patients referred. The team's work now extends into many aspects of chronic non-malignant disease management, ethical decision making, and increasing involvement with children.

Codes of practice

Palliative care teams need to interact frequently with other professional teams. The interface needs to be managed carefully to be successful. It involves negotiation, good communication, mutual respect and understanding. The code of practice we agreed at the outset to deal with this has proved to be satisfactory over a number of years. For hospital patient referrals, the consultant team who are caring for the patient must consent to the referral. For a patient living at home, referral to the palliative care team must have the consent of the GP. Also, if a patient dies under our care, the GP must be notified within an hour. The local medical committee agreed to this so that messages could be relayed to relevant doctors via the deputising and answering services. It has avoided the problem of GPs visiting distressed relatives without being aware of a death.

When seeing patients in hospital or in their own homes we always act as invited guests. Our role is to advise and not to take over care, so tact and negotiating skills are required to ensure that nobody is undermined and that patient care is optimised. Team building, supporting clinical teams and reducing feelings of isolation are all part of our daily work.

Healthcare is increasingly defined by boundaries. These may arise between different trusts, because of contracts, where charities impose limits, and where different departments may be subject to competition and rivalry. Such boundaries need to be crossed in the interest of patient care. Age and diagnosis are no bar to our initial involvement but we may refer cases on to others who may be better resourced and have expertise to offer. The age range of patients referred is 18 months to 102 years with a median of 65.4 years. We liaise with all local agencies and are working towards core documentation to defined roles clearly and avoid overlap and duplication.

Ethical decision making

The principles of autonomy, beneficence, non-maleficence and justice are well-defined, but, in palliative care, ethical dilemmas are common. A feeding gastrostomy might give benefit in motor neurone disease, but severe communication difficulties may raise doubts about the patient's ability to consent to or refuse the procedure. It may be correct to withhold treatments or abandon resuscitation attempts in those where the outlook is hopeless, as in those with severe brain damage from trauma, but the decision is often made with anxiety and sadness. The recent increase in advance directives, or living wills, however well they have been drawn up, seems to have increased the need for advice on ethical principles. The House of Lords Report on Medical Ethics[2] has been helpful. It makes it clear that the doctor has a duty to undertake treatments that enhance the patient as a person and that futile treatments should be considered unjustified.

Children and parents

A difficulty facing any sick parent is what the children should be told, and this may depend upon their maturity. For convenience, children's psychological development may be divided into three stages according to their understanding of life-threatening disease and death. Those under 5 years of age see the world in very ego-centric terms, and concepts of time and finality have little meaning. Life and death may almost seem interchangeable, with dead simply meaning less alive. Children are often preoccupied by questions of what happens to a dead body, for example whether it can still hear or whether it would feel the heat in the crematorium.

In the primary school years of about 5–8 years, death itself can assume the identity of a frightening person, so that it is the lucky ones who escape. Children are now aware of the terrible finality of death and their interest focuses on the rituals surrounding it. The media constantly remind them that violence and aggression are associated with sudden death, but the slow death from disease, typically depicted in 19th and early 20th century paintings, is unfamiliar to children today.

Over the age of about 8 years children's concepts are as sophisticated as adults'. Death is final, irreversible and universal. They may feel shame at having unhealthy parents, the disease somehow tainting those close to it. They are often very practical and clear in their concerns, wanting to care and show love, but being acutely sensitive to taboos imposed by adults. All too often these children are excluded from key dialogues. They may hide their anxieties for fear of making things worse than they are already.

Children's responses to the illness or death of a parent or sibling, and their level of knowledge and understanding, are easily underestimated. They seem acutely aware of what is going on[3,4] and may be more sensitive to the atmosphere than the adults around them. They may want to sit by their dying parent, be present at the moment of death, and attend the funeral.

We now offer a bereavement service for children and adolescents, whether or not the deceased was known to our centre. The greatest regret that children voice after the death of a parent is often that they did not know the gravity of the illness. Because of this, they did not take the opportunity to show their love. Instead, they may remember angry terms used by the parent, like 'You'll be the death of me' and thus carry a burden of guilt, believing that they have, in some way, caused the illness.

Parents facing death, especially if they are single, may need help to arrange continuing care for their children. They may wish to leave letters to be opened by their children on their 18th, 21st and other key birthdays. These may affirm their love and remind of things that made this child so special. Such communications are deeply personal, but dying parents can gain peace from a sense of completion of a life task. Within the concept of holistic care for the patient, these do become medical and nursing issues.

The arrival of genetic markers for disease has brought its own problems for families. Where there is an unfavourable family history, the breast cancer gene[5] has caused more anxiety for mothers who have daughters. This is particularly frustrating at present, as there is still no effective way of predicting the disease in the individuals at risk.

Conclusion

The best thing we can do for the dying person is to strive to provide optimum care and ensure a peaceful death, with support to those who are bereaved. The care of patients extends beyond death to the provision of bereavement services. We are now able to offer a service to the newly bereaved and, if they wish, an introduction to a support group for the young and the adult.

References

1. Tarr S, Roberts DE, Spencer MG, Tarr MJ, Finlay I. Symptom control of cancer patients at a teaching hospital. *Pharmaceutical Journal* 1992; **249**: R43.

2. Walton JN. *House of Lords Select Committee on Medical Ethics.* London: HMSO, 1995.

3. Bluebond-Langner M. The private worlds of dying children. Oxford: Princeton University Press, 1978.

4. Jewett Cl. Helping children cope with separation and loss. London: Batsford, 1994.

5. Evans DGR, Fentiman IS, McPherson K, Ashbury D, Ponder BA, Howell A. Familial breast cancer. *British Medical Journal* 1994; **308**: 183–7.

9 Terminal illness and the family

Barbara Monroe

Director of Social Work, St Christopher's Hospice, London

Terminal illness has an impact on the patient at many levels: physical health, independence, career and status, predictability, future plans, motivation and meaning. A diagnosis of terminal illness also affects the family, threatening the stable pattern of relating which most families develop over time. The patient's loss of self confidence may be experienced in parallel by their families and friends. Professional attention to potential difficulties in family life can help to mitigate negative consequences.

Impact of terminal illness on the family

The effects of terminal illness on the family are largely independent of the diagnosis. For example, they are similar for cancer, motor neurone disease, multiple sclerosis, renal failure, heart disease or chronic obstructive airways disease. By the time the medical journey is coming to an end with terminal care, the family and patient will have seen a series of different professionals who will all have told them different things at different times. Uncertainty and the ambiguity of the transition to palliative care may have added to the feelings of helplessness already engendered by the patient's physical deterioration. All these factors may well have led to a breakdown in communication in the patient's family.[1]

The patient and family will be experiencing role changes, practical changes, such as the loss of employment and decreased finances, social isolation and physical exhaustion. There will be the sense of loss of control and privacy as life is invaded by outsiders. In addition, everyone will be facing the personal confusion and anguish of powerful, unexpected and conflicting feelings. Above all there will be a pervasive sense of anxiety and fear. The juice will have been squeezed out of life.

Under these pressures, the patient and family may retreat into fear and denial, individuals holding on to agonizing burdens and distancing themselves from one another when they most need support and intimacy. They will all want to protect others and themselves from further hurt, particularly if professionals imply that the truth is too dangerous to share. The work of specialist palliative care units with cancer patients and their families has helped us to understand what assists the majority of families to face such problems.[2]

Meeting the family

Terminal illness tends to be experienced in the home so dying is a family affair. The unit of care often needs to be the patient within the family. Meeting the family can give us information about the patient within the context of a community within society. The entire social network contains resources which can be marshalled to help meet the consequences of illness and death. Professionals who ignore the family may overlook all sorts of benefits. Making the family part of the caring team offers the possibility of encouraging and using their strengths and resources rather than simply cataloguing the difficulties they face. Failure to involve and support them may increase the need for residential care if family care breaks down.

For some families, good palliative care may also become effective preventive health care. The way professionals help a family to manage illness and death may have a profound impact on both their health in bereavement and their capacity to cope with other emotional crises.

Without sensitivity, professionals may impose further losses upon the family. They may be anxious that seeing the patient and family together may take too long or get out of control. They may feel helpless and fear blame from the family. Seeing families reminds us that patients are people and this increases the risk that their problems could touch us personally.

Continuity of professional care is necessary if people are to develop a sense of trust. Co-ordination is important if the family is not to feel swamped and confused. Too little help reduces options; too much, delivered by a whole range of concerned and worried professionals, can leave a family exhausted, de-skilled, and convinced that problems are beyond resolution. The mother of a dying child spoke of the time absorbed by the visits, and the sometimes conflicting advice of a GP, district nurse, Macmillan nurse, health visitor and hospital psychologist. She said despairingly: 'I need to do it my way'. Professionals can also make the wrong assumptions about what the patient and family need to hear, and when. Some of these will be based on cultural misunderstanding.[3]

To make family care successful, the task of the professional is to support, not to protect. For example, it is not necessarily to relieve sadness, but to support people whilst they experience it. To explain the diagnosis and treatment is not enough, we need to explore the meaning of events for the patient and family.

The task of specialist palliative care units should include the development of clear and effective tools[4] which will assist non-specialists to deliver quality care. The challenge is to make our findings appropriate to the majority of the patient population, their families and their professional carers. There is also a need for methods to identify the few complex or high risk families which will need specialist help, perhaps from a social worker, psychologist, or specialist palliative care unit.

Faced with a dying patient within a family, the task of any professional is apparent. There needs to be a clear and adequate flow of information at a speed acceptable to them, and there must be adequate opportunity for questions to be asked. Emotional pain should be acknowledged and ways found of allowing it to be expressed and shared. Unfamiliar emotions often demand reassurance. The family may need support in deciding which goals are important and realistic, and how they might be achieved.

Assessing need

The palliative care approach necessary for most families can be provided by the medical team already caring for the patient. A clear family assessment will also give information about the necessary extent and locus of family support. Its main perspectives are the patient, the family and their physical and social resources.

Most families we meet want to say important things to one another, to plan for the future and to be involved in care. They may be overwhelmed by an unfamiliar situation, not knowing how to begin and what to say, so a little help may go a long way. Lack of information leaves people at the mercy of their fears and fantasies. Many will want to know how the illness is likely to progress, how difficult symptoms will be treated and what practical help will be available. Without such information planning is impossible. A single meeting of the whole family, made safe by the presence of a neutral professional, where thoughts can be shared and questions asked together, may release a family's capacity for action.

The assessment should clarify the fears and aims of the patient, identify the ways in which life has changed and discern who is providing support. It should reveal the normal coping mechanisms of the family, gauge the impact of the illness on close partnerships, detect other changes or difficulties in the family and identify other

vulnerable individuals. It should give awareness of the family's eth-
nic, cultural and religious background and the formal and informal
helping systems in the social environment.

Unmet physical needs should be explored: a washing machine,
additional financial benefits, aids to daily living, a volunteer sitter, a
day centre place, or a holiday grant may avoid or delay the need for
in-patient care. Such issues can become the biggest concerns of the
patient and family, particularly over a long and exhausting illness.

Talking with families

Professionals can provide an opportunity for families to share their
anxieties and begin to achieve compromises. Families are often
reassured to discover that, although their situation is unique, they
are not alone and that what they are facing has been experienced by
others. A wife, looking after a husband disabled by stroke, may be
relieved to know that she is neither mad nor bad to sometimes wish
him dead. We know the sorts of questions which help people to
explore their feelings and explain themselves to one another:

- What worries you most about the illness?
- What is helping most at present?
- What else would help you to cope?
- What else do you need to know about your illness or treat-
  ment?
- What is the worst thing at the moment?

Confirming what can be done, giving information about what
usually happens and what the options are, can help the family to
exercise choice and reassert its own sense of worth by making
decisions.

Children

Care offered to the family is incomplete without considering the
needs of children. Exclusion carries a price.[5] A child under the age
of 10 years who loses a parent has a roughly doubled chance of
depressive illness in adulthood. This probability is moderated by the
amount of information available to the child at the time of the
death and the support received both at that time and subsequently.
There is a tendency for adults to consider it a matter of choice
whether or not children should become involved in the issues of

terminally illness. Of course, it is impossible not to communicate.[6] Children are aware of changes in routine, they read the emotions around them, they respond to body language and they overhear conversations. They quickly sense when something so important is happening in their family. In our desire to protect children we may succeed in isolating them, excluding them from family concerns and leaving them alone with their fantasies.

Children cannot ultimately be protected from the truth. They will be sad. The task is to offer them support in their sadness, and to do this we have to help their parents to help them. There are good reasons why parents sometimes resist involving their children. They may not know what their children understand about illness and death or what words to use. They themselves will be grieving and will be anxious about their ability to maintain control. Professionals can help by giving them advice about explanations of illness appropriate to their child's age and about the kinds of reactions they may anticipate. Lists of suitable books and leaflets can be provided for parents to read with their children. Some parents welcome talking to their children with a professional present.[7] Just one such meeting may give them confidence to continue for themselves. Parents may also need help to involve other people, such as teachers or friends.

Children need information, reassurance, a chance to express their feelings[8] and to have their loss acknowledged. They will also need adults who share their feelings. Children learn to grieve and to face loss by observing others. They are often uncertain about what is allowed and need to see the reactions of others, especially their parents.

Bereavement care

Specialist palliative care units have a responsibility to help general hospitals to develop packages of bereavement care that are realistic in terms of time and resources. Bereavement begins before the death of a patient and much can be achieved by providing help in advance. Professionals need to help families to create good enough memories for the future. The family will need to feel that whilst the patient was alive they did what they could to help. Discussions should be held about whether or not each individual wishes to be present at the time of death. There is a need to know how symptoms will be controlled and what will happen immediately after death, so that undue fears will not determine decisions. Family members can be offered the opportunity to help wash and dress the body if they wish, and deference must be paid to practices required by religion and culture. It is important to remember the part that any death will play in the grieving of other patients and their families. They too need to be told promptly and sensitively that the death has occurred.

Much can be achieved by a single, brief visit or meeting shortly after the death. This may encourage and answer questions about the illness and death and also reinforce the reality of the death, for example with an opportunity to view the body, to read the death certificate and to deal with returned property. At the same time, practical advice can be offered about the funeral. Most importantly, it allows the family care of the patient to be validated and permits thanks and farewells for both family and staff.

Whatever the pressures on a particular unit, all families might be given simple leaflets about grieving which include telephone numbers of local bereavement services. Grief is not an illness and most people will manage it with the help of their family, friends and social network. Even so, the use of risk assessment guidelines may help hospitals to identify those individuals who might be actively assisted to seek bereavement counselling.[9] In addition many hospitals now recognise the value of providing ritual grieving opportunities such as memorial services.

Improving and extending palliative care

Attention to detail may upgrade care from good to excellent. In hospitals, simple methods of making the family welcome and paying them attention are all part of good care. A formal opportunity for the family to meet with a member of staff, and clear written information about the hospital, the particular ward, its facilities and personnel, all reduce anxiety caused by lack of familiarity. Written information about the illness and sources of help need to be available in languages appropriate to the local community.

Hospital staff need access to a range of specialist information. They need to know about resources in the local community, such as twilight nurses. Risk assessment tools may help them to decide who should be contacted in bereavement and who would benefit from referral to the psychologist or social worker. Simple protocols might define what should be provided for families after a death, and to what financial benefits are people entitled.

Hospital links with primary health care teams need to work effectively. There is still a tendency for patients to be discharged from hospital to their families, having received unco-ordinated care from a number of specialist teams. This might be resolved by a variety of methods. There needs to be a key worker. Shared documentation also helps to make professional communication co-ordinated, consistent and understandable to the patient.

Specialist units can influence standards of palliative care by example, educational initiatives and research. The educational approach for doctors and nurses should begin in their training before qualification. It should continue in the workplace where, by adaptation of specialist palliative expertise to local requirements, it becomes part of the fabric of good care.

Courses organised by specialist palliative care units allow professionals to train in a specific subject and then act as an expert resource for the rest of their team. Such courses might deal with issues of sexuality or working with children.

Relevant research in the field of palliative care includes the prudent use of resources. Attempts are being made to measure the impact of respite care nursing packages on numbers of home deaths and the value of staff support programmes[10] in improving family care. Consultancy services are under development for non-malignant disease and earlier stages of cancer. Professional helplines give rapid access to a multidisciplinary telephone advisory service. Specialist resources such as groups for bereaved children or lone fathers can be extended to local GPs, schools and hospitals. Written materials are being developed such as a simple bereavement leaflet designed specifically for children.[11]

The palliative approach to family care is relevant to anyone who comes into contact with advanced disease or its broader consequences. We have recently run training programmes for the Police on breaking bad news, for staff in the Department of Social Security on helping bereaved relatives, and for schools on managing loss in the classroom.

Conclusion

We do know what helps most patients and their families as they face incurable illness. Specialist palliative care teams have a responsibility to provide fellow professionals with clear descriptions of concrete and effective packages of care. They need to encourage the use of appropriate tools for the psycho-social care of the majority. They also need to develop reliable methods to identify the complex few who should then have access to specialist palliative care, whatever their disease status.

Specialist palliative care teams need to continue to emphasise the importance of self knowledge and experiential training. Working with loss reminds us of our own previous losses and of those we fear in the future. We need to feel comfortable about this if we are to be truly effective.

References

1. Kirschling JM (ed). Family-based palliative care. New York: Howarth Press, 1990.

2. Monroe B. Psychosocial dimensions of palliation. In Saunders C, Sykes N (eds). The management of terminal malignant disease. Edition 3. London: Edward Arnold, 1993; 174–201.

3. Oliviere D. Cross-cultural principles of care. In: Saunders C, Sykes N (eds). The management of terminal malignant disease. Edition 3. London: Edward Arnold, 1993; 202–12.

4. Vachon M, Kristjanson L, Higginson I. Psychosocial issues in palliative care: the patient, the family and the process and outcome of care. *Journal of Pain and Symptom Management* 1995; **10**: 142–50.

5. Black D. The bereaved child. *Journal of Child Psychology and Psychiatry* 1978; **19**: 287–92.

6. Monroe B. Helping the grieving family. In: Smith S, Pennells M (eds). Interventions with bereaved children. London, Jessica Kingsley, 1995; 87–106.

7. Hildebrand J. Working with a bereaved family. *Palliative Medicine* 1989; **3**: 105–11.

8. Hemmings P. Working with children facing bereavement as individuals. *European Journal of Palliative Care* 1994; **1**: 72-7.

9. Sanders C. Risk factors in bereavement outcome. In: Stroebe M, Stroebe W, Hansson R (eds). *Handbook of bereavement: theory research and intervention.* New York: Cambridge University Press, 1993: 255-67.

10. Vachon M. Occupational stress in the care of the critically ill, the dying and the bereaved. Washington: Hemisphere, 1987.

11. St Christopher's Hospice. Someone special has died. London: St Christopher's Hospice, 1989.

Marie Curie Cancer Care — its aims and work

Marie Curie Cancer Care (formerly the Marie Curie Memorial Foundation) was created in 1948 with a mission towards patients with cancer. In 1952, a needs survey of 7,000 patients with cancer underlined the lack of services for those living at home and led to the setting up of the Marie Curie Nursing Service. Since that time Marie Curie Cancer Care has grown into the most comprehensive and diverse cancer charity in the UK.

Marie Curie Centres

Marie Curie Cancer Care now offers specialist palliative care in its eleven hospice centres, with 290 beds and a range of home care, day care, outpatient services including lymphoedema clinics and bereavement services. Its 290 inpatient beds amount to approximately 11% of the hospice beds in the voluntary sector throughout the UK. Almost all of the Marie Curie centres are consultant led and it is expected that by the end of 1996 there will be more than 20 consultants employed in the eleven centres, all of whom also have NHS contracts. The centres play an appropriate part in training medical, nursing and other staff in specialist palliative care.

Marie Curie Nursing Service

Marie Curie's national network of nurses gives over a million hours of hands on care in patients' own homes as needed and without charge — overnight or throughout the day. The service is available 365 days a year. Marie Curie nurses care for almost 40% of patients at home with late-stage cancer and their work complements that of the district nursing service and primary health care team. Marie Curie nurses are selected for their knowledge and interest in the subject of palliative care nursing and all grades (nursing auxiliary, enrolled nurses and registered general nurses) have induction and continuing education programmes.

Education

Marie Curie Cancer Care from the start recognised the importance of public education about cancer and the need for the best possible training for staff, both in its own hospice centres and those working in the cancer field, whether in prevention, active treatment or palliative care. It has an active and innovative education department in London which organises local, regional and national courses and conferences as well as fostering training and education based on the eleven hospice centres.

Research

The internationally recognised Marie Curie Research Institute at Oxted, Surrey, is directed towards the search for genetic keys to the prevention and cure of cancer. Recently, Marie Curie Cancer Care has set up an additional funding arrangement coupled with education and training in the field of palliative care research with the objective of ensuring that service and teaching are increasingly research based.

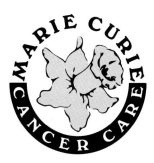

Marie Curie Cancer Care

28 Belgrave Square
London
SW1X 8QG

Tel: 0171 235 3325
Fax: 0171 823 2380